"Paula Squires paints a sensitive and nuanced portrait of a truly different kind of man: Donald Bridges Jr. His embrace of the totality of his life—despite its many challenges and obstacles—serves as a reminder that true strength comes from deep within. When he declares, "I'm still here. There must be a reason," Donald boldly begins a lifelong journey to find the answer. Along the way, he touches many lives and provides hope in the face of despair. As one friend marvels, "I've learned... there's nothing in life, with God's help, that you can't overcome."

— CHIP JONES,
author of *The Organ Thieves: The Shocking Story
of the First Heart Transplant in the Segregated South*,
winner of the Library of Virginia 2021 Literary Award for Nonfiction

"...There are far too many accounts of the ways disability can change your life for the worse, and far too few accounts about the virtues of disability: the things that disability teaches an individual and, hopefully as a result, those around that individual about the strength and imagination of the human spirit, and what it means to truly live with courage. In *A Different Kind of Courage*, Paula Squires adds to the voices of people looking to change the way disability is represented and, therefore, understood. Through chronicling the life of the remarkable Donald Bridges, we can better understand how the lives of people with disabilities are valuable, important, and to be celebrated."

—BROOKE ELLISON,
associate professor of health policy and medical ethics,
Stony Brook University,
and author of *Miracles Happen and Look Both Ways*

"Many people around the world are sitting in wheelchairs or in beds waiting for a glimpse of hope. *In A Different Kind of Courage*, Paula Squires provides that hope by sharing the inspirational story of how one man survived a spinal cord injury. His courage in the face of devastating injury coupled with Squires' reporting on the latest adaptive technologies highlights what is a new era in the field of spinal cord injury. Today, people can see the path of hope shining, and some are declaring victory over paralysis."

— ASHRAF GORGEY,
director of spinal cord injury research, Central Virginia VA Health Care System

"*A Different Kind of Courage* should be at the top of anyone's reading list who values seeing life from a different perspective. Paula Squires gives the able-bodied reader an intimate look into every facet of Donald Bridges Jr.'s life following a traumatic spinal cord injury. So often, success in spinal cord injuries is measured by, and celebrated, when a paralyzed individual regains the ability to walk. Squires offers the often-untold success stories of the other 96% who adapt and go on to live rewarding lives from the wheelchair level; becoming graduates, starting careers, falling in love, raising children—all the things people celebrate no matter their circumstances. As an individual living with quadriplegia, and who works with individuals living with spinal cord injuries, I wholeheartedly appreciate the lengths that Squires and Bridges have gone to give folks a better understanding of how people live with spinal cord injuries and what it takes to get there."

— RICHARD BAGBY,
executive director, United Spinal Association of Virginia

COURAGE

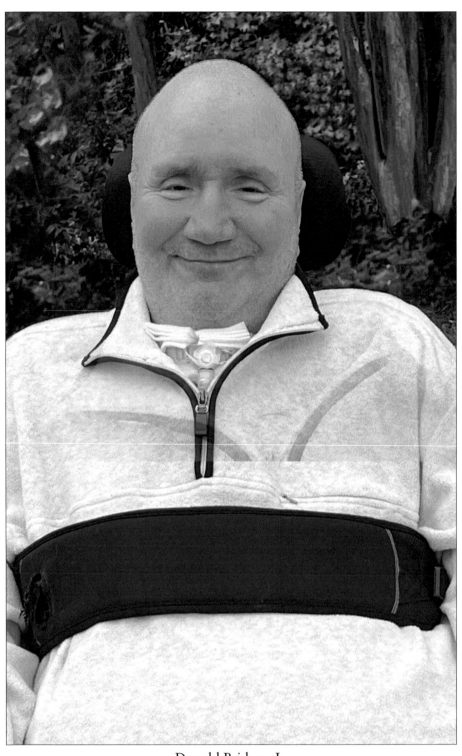

Donald Bridges, Jr.

A DIFFERENT KIND OF
COURAGE

*One Man's Story of Triumph
Over Paralysis*

by

PAULA C. SQUIRES

DEMENTI MILESTONE PUBLISHING

Author
Paula C. Squires

Publisher
Wayne Dementi
Dementi Milestone Publishing, Inc.
Manakin-Sabot, VA 23103
www.dementimilestonepublishing
Cataloging-in-publication data for this book is available from
The Library of Congress.
ISBN: 979-8-9856150-6-7

Graphic design by:
Jayne E. Hushen
Dementi Milestone Publishing, Inc.

Printed in the U.S.A.

Attempts have been made to identify the owners of any copyrighted materials appearing in this book. The publisher extends his apology for any
errors or omissions and encourages copyright owners inadvertently missed
to contact him.

DEDICATION

For Dean, a champion of the underdog.

CONTENTS

INTRODUCTION

More than three decades ago, while working as a reporter for the *Richmond Times-Dispatch* in Richmond, Virginia, I met an extraordinary young man. His name was Donald "Don" Bridges Jr.

Don dislocated his neck while playing rugby and was paralyzed from the neck down. He had just returned home following rehabilitation at an out-of-state hospital. My assignment was to describe how a middle-class family was coping with the catastrophic injury of its only son.

I was nervous about meeting Don, my first interview with a severely disabled person. His parents told me he would be in a wheelchair and hooked up to a ventilator. When Don entered the room, the sound of the ventilator was the first thing I heard: a soft, constant whoosh as the machine gave him a breath, enabling him to speak.

I stood stiffly, trying not to show how taken aback I was at the sight of this handsome, athletic-built young man. Don had broad shoulders, dark hair, and a tentative smile. At 25, he was a quadriplegic, unable to walk, dress or feed himself.

As we chatted about his daily routine, Don teased me when I mistakenly thought he said the ventilator supplied him with 10 breaths an hour, rather than 10 breaths a minute. "I'd be kind of blue, wouldn't I?"

Don's humor and self-deprecating nature put me at

ease. They have been important allies in his long journey with paralysis, but that's getting ahead of the story.

Many people don't survive an injury like Don's. Some of the ones who do sink into a deep depression at the thought of being tied to a wheelchair for the rest of their lives. Don did not speak with bitterness about his injury. He focused on the challenges of rebuilding his life.

"There are still a lot of things I want to do," he told me. "I'm going to try and do them."

I was struck by Don's courage. Life as he had known it had been irrevocably altered, and his future was uncertain. Yet, he was rising to the challenge of a new normal. The rigors of the battlefield require physical courage. Moral courage requires people to take a stand, sometimes at great risk to themselves or others. Don summoned a different kind of courage, an inner strength that bubbled up like a mountain spring, nourishing his soul so he wouldn't give in to despair.

"At 25, I wasn't ready to die," Don said. Instead, with steely resolve, Don found the will to endure.

The headline on the story that ran in the *Times-Dispatch* on March 13, 1988, reflected Don's life-affirming outlook: "I have more good days than bad."

The story stayed with me for a long time. On Monday mornings, when I grumbled about going to work, I would think about Don and how he grieved the loss of simple things like throwing off the covers and getting out of bed.

Over the years we stayed in touch. I wrote other stories

about Don's progress. Today, after 35 years of paralysis, he is one of the longest living, ventilator-dependent quadriplegics in the country. As we have been reminded during a long pandemic, anyone's life can change in an instant. Don's journey is instructive for all; not only because it shines a light into the life of the disabled—how they live and how they cope—but also as a testimony to the resilience of the human spirit and the power of community as Don forges a new path with dignity and grace.

Journalism taught me the power of shared experience. Don agreed to share his story in the hope that it might help others.

Paula C. Squires

PROLOGUE

Past Meets Present

The first thing Don noticed as he maneuvered his wheelchair through the sliding glass doors was the vibe. Sunlight streamed through a four-story glass atrium, bathing the lobby in light. It provided a dramatic setting for an overhead sculpture. Down at eye level colorful banners welcomed visitors. When he stopped at the registration desk, Don felt like he was checking into an upscale hotel instead of a hospital tour.

The tour's first stop, off the lobby, was a 10,000-square-foot gym. This was grand central for patients as they put in their required three hours of physical therapy a day. The goal? Get damaged muscles moving again.

An overhead tracking system made it possible for staff to slip people into harnesses, giving them full body-weight support as they practiced the motions of walking. Don marveled at the technology. Back when he underwent physical rehabilitation, he laid on a gym floor while physical therapists moved his limbs through a range of motions.

Today's toolbox of therapies was light years ahead. Some of the machines massaged muscles with electrical stimulation. A patient could even go bionic via a robotic exoskeleton. The battery-powered skeleton could be strapped to the legs and trunks of paralyzed people, enabling them to take steps.

The next stop, the hospital's spinal-cord injury unit, was also impressive. Every room was equipped with a large plasma television that could be turned on via a mouth-operated sip and puff command. Voice activation controls were coming soon, said a nurse. Helpful tools, thought Don, since a remote is useless for someone paralyzed from the neck down.

After living with paralysis for more than three decades, who better than Don to compare how far things had come in the world of the spinal cord injured?

As he wheeled his way outside into the spring sunshine, the balmy weather reminded Don of the day when his life changed in an instant.

Part One

Life Interrupted

1

'Organized Mayhem'

The day began like most Saturdays, with Don gathering his gear for a rugby match. His team, the James River Rugby Football Club, was playing its arch local rival, the R.A.T.S (Richmond Area Training Side). They were rats all right, thought Don, remembering the previous fall when the R.A.T.S knocked Don's team out of the state championship playoffs during the first game. With sunny skies and temperatures in the 70s, the May weather was perfect for a rematch.

Don's girlfriend, Patty Sgueglia, would be cheering him on. He met her on a blind date, and the two clicked. After more than a year of dating, the couple was getting serious, talking about marriage once Don completed his graduate degree.

Springtime in Virginia is glorious with dogwood trees and azaleas in full bloom. So, too, was this season of Don's life. His whole future stretched before him, full of possibility.

Don was working his way through a graduate program in health administration at Richmond's Medical College of Virginia (MCV). Taking classes and working at the hospital kept him busy, so he welcomed the chance to get outside on Saturday for a weekly rugby match. An only child, he thrived on the comradery of the rugby team.

He started playing rugby on a club team during his senior year at Virginia Tech. He played various positions, mostly on the second row—"anything to get on the field," he said. After college, Don returned to his hometown of Richmond, Virginia, and played club rugby for two seasons for the R.A.T.S before leaving for James River. Don switched teams because the R.A.T.S didn't take winning seriously. "It was more of a social thing," he said. "The team's motto seemed to be, 'Let's go do something on the field and then go out and party.'"

James River was a more competitive club. Formed in 1969, it was one of the oldest clubs in the region, with a roster of experienced players. "I wanted to be a part of it."

Rugby, along with American football, is a full-contact sport. Unlike football, though, with compulsory helmets and pads, rugby players aren't required to wear protective gear aside from a mouthpiece. To mitigate the danger of head and neck injuries, players can't tackle someone above the shoulders.

At six feet and 180 pounds, Don played the position of hooker, one of the team's forwards. He had played hooker for the R.A.T.S and was now playing the same position for

James River because that's where the team had an opening. "When I got to Richmond, no one wanted to play hooker. It wasn't my favorite position," he told friends, "but I thought I was pretty decent at it."

Hookers see most of their action during a scrum. The formation is called to restart a game following minor infractions. Some fans go wild for scrums because they offer a display of raw, brute strength. Picture a group of grown men grunting and pushing at each other with all their might.

A scrum forms when eight forwards from each team face off against each other. Each side forms into three rows. Players crouch nearly to the ground, lower their heads and lock arms around one another's shoulders. Then the two sides push in what is known as "binding in."

According to some studies, this battle is the equivalent of exerting 3,700 pounds of force. As the No. 2. forward on the front line, the hooker plays a key position, in the middle of the scrum.

As the packs come together, the ball is rolled through a gap—called the tunnel—between the two teams. It's the hooker's job to gain possession by hooking the ball backward with his feet, a tough assignment, with people pushing at you from both directions. It's no wonder some sports writers refer to rugby as "organized mayhem."

When Don arrived at the field that day, "There was a lot of rivalry," he said. This was the first time James River was facing the R.A.T.S since the loss in the fall. During that game, Don played hooker for James River. He didn't want to lose again. Neither did James River Rugby coach and co-captain Mike Toney. Nicknamed "crazy legs," because of his ability to run and make cuts, Toney played No. 6 as wing forward.

"I gave a great big pep talk before the game, saying it was a fluke we lost to them in the first place ... We are going to avenge this loss," Toney told the team.

The R.A.T.S had a reputation for playing a tough, physical game. One of Don's teammates, Pat Grover, was a paramedic who volunteered for the local rescue squad. He invited some of the squad members, including his girlfriend, to come to the game that day to cheer for James River. They parked their ambulance on the street by the field.

2

The Scrum

Don and his teammates arrived at the field at noon for warmups before the 1 p.m. game. Terry Byrd, who played the No. 8 position as a back forward, watched as Don chased his girlfriend around the sidelines. Byrd was the player who returned the ball to play after Don moved it to the back of the scrum. As the game got underway, "We were playing well," said Byrd. So were the R.A.T.S, making a score.

In the first 20 minutes, three scrums were called. Don successfully hooked the ball for his team. "I easily won the put in of the ball the first three times."

Then a fourth scrum was called. "When we went in, they weren't ready; we weren't ready. We sort of butted heads and backed up. The ref called it," said Toney.

"When we engaged for the second time, Don didn't quite get in as he needed to, and he tried to force himself in," recalled Toney. "Once Don got his head and neck in, then our team pushed and drove completely over the other team."

Don remembers that the two teams came together forcibly. "That's illegal. It's called barging. You're supposed to come together in a controlled manner, not real hard."

This time the ref didn't blow his whistle. Meanwhile, "I didn't get my head down in time." Don said his forehead, rather than his shoulder, lodged into the shoulder of an opposing player. "I immediately felt pain in my neck."

After the scrum released, everyone moved off to play—everyone except Don.

He crashed to the ground. "I was lying flat on my back, looking up at the sky. My body felt like it was somewhere else. I felt a burning sensation in the back of my neck and was having a hard time breathing."

Toney saw Don and rushed to his side. "Are you okay?"

Gasping for air, Don responded, "I can't breathe."

Byrd knew something was wrong because Don hadn't hooked for the ball. "When we went in, his leg went limp. I'm like, 'Why in the hell didn't he hook?' We lost the ball. They got it. I was a little upset. Then I saw him. He was pretty much in the fetal position. He couldn't breathe. That's when I knew something wasn't right. Then I went from upset to panicking."

Toney yelled at Grover. "Get over here!"

Grover rushed over and knew immediately that Don's

injury was severe. He called his girlfriend over, and she intubated Don, putting a tube into his mouth and down his trachea. That created a direct route into the lungs, so Don could breathe by being attached to a supply of oxygen.

By then, Byrd, Toney and Grover were screaming for help. The rescue squad members sprang into action, carrying Don off the field and putting him into the ambulance, before driving to MCV, a short distance away in downtown Richmond. While the rest of the team knew Don was injured, they didn't know the severity of the injury. Grover suspected Don had dislocated his neck.

Sgueglia remembers seeing Don drop on the field. "They didn't let me run to him."

After the game resumed, "We went on to destroy that team. We beat them very bad, 40 to something … The game had to go on," said Toney. As soon as it ended, everyone wanted to know, "'How's Don?' We had all been playing rugby for years and had never seen anyone get hurt, so it was sort of a freak thing."

As the team's coach, he was the one who assigned Don to play hooker. "He was a good player, and he was happy to do it," said Toney. Yet, it was a call he would second guess for the rest of his life. When Toney called Don's dad at the hospital to check on his teammate, "He said, 'Don's neck is completely broken.'"

3

Calm Before the Storm

E llen Bridges had been married to Don's father,
Donald H. Bridges (who the family calls Don Sr. to
distinguish between the two), for slightly more than a year
when they got the call about Don's injury on Saturday,
May 2, 1987. "We were just putting the finishing touches
on some landscaping in our front yard when Don's girlfriend, Patty, called. She said Donnie had been injured playing rugby. She said he couldn't move or breathe. I immediately knew that this was a life-altering event. Don Sr. and I
changed our clothes and raced to the emergency room. On
the way there, I wondered if Donnie would survive."

Don's dad also remembers the call. "They said, 'You
need to get to the hospital now.'"

When the couple arrived, an attendant took them back
to see Don. "He was on a table that appeared to be in an
X-ray room. I'm not sure if he was conscious at the time,"
recalled Don Sr. "It was hard for me to see Don."

Patty said she called people all afternoon from the hospital's pay phone. "I wasn't allowed to see him because I wasn't a family member."

The doctors told the family that Don was lucky to be alive. Had paramedics not been on hand to provide immediate emergency care, Don would have died on the field. The impact from a split second in the scrum dislocated his neck and severed his spinal cord between the C3 and C4 cervical vertebra. Doctors at MCV immediately performed a high-risk surgery to stabilize his injured spinal cord. Doctors told Don Sr. that "the spinal cord is like a tube of toothpaste. Once you pull it apart, you can't get it back together again with all the same connections."

In other words, his only son would be a quadriplegic who would never walk again. The situation seemed surreal. Just when Don Sr.'s life was going in a positive direction with a new marriage, his son's life seemed to hang in the balance. This was the kid who played football in high school, who loved to fish and hunt and now he was paralyzed in all four limbs. Don Sr. struggled to accept his son's bleak future. "Why does something like that happen to someone?"

Yet Don Jr. already was showing determination to rise above his catastrophic injury. "He wanted to live from the word go," said Don Sr. "I couldn't believe a psychologist at the hospital kept asking him, 'Do you want to live?' Don's emphatic reply: "Yes."

Dr. Kevin Keller also got the call about Don. Don had worked for Dr. Keller as part of his front office staff for about a year and half before Keller left a family practice in Colonial Heights for another family practice nearby. Keller had just returned home from church and heard his phone ringing.

"I picked up the phone and there was this hysterical woman, screaming and crying. I had to ask her to please calm down because I couldn't understand what she was saying. It was Don's mother, Jutta. She was trying to tell me that he had broken his neck."

Keller immediately drove to MCV. He hadn't seen Don since leaving Colonial Heights six months before. The doctor was fond of this athletic graduate student who'd show up for work on Mondays with a bandage on his face or arm as a result of playing rugby. Through the years, Don had broken his nose numerous times as well.

When Keller arrived at the hospital, "It was horrible. Donnie was lying in bed. They had the halo on him where they tried to secure his neck. When I saw him, he wouldn't open his eyes. I was talking with him, and a tear came out of the corner of his eye. I remember kissing him on the forehead."

A medical halo is a metal ring attached to a patient's head to stabilize the spine. It's held in place by a series of pins equally spaced around the ring. Don could feel sensations from the neck up, and he remembers when the medical team placed the halo's metal crown on his head. "It was ironic since this resident kept asking me if I felt this pinprick or that pinprick, and I said, 'No.' Then they put the halo on, and I said, 'I felt that.'"

The sharp stab was the last thing Don remembered for a

week. "My best guess is that it was too much to take in, so my brain shut down."

Exactly one week to the day after Don dislocated his neck, he woke up in the hospital and saw a nurse in his room.

"Hey buddy, how are you doing?" she inquired.

"I looked at her and was thinking 'Who are you? Where am I?'"

Now that he was awake, he could hear it: the beep of a ventilator, pumping air into his lungs. With spinal cord injuries, just a few inches make a difference. A break in the C5 to C6 cervical vertebrae means a person will be in a wheelchair but will probably have use of his arms and be able to breathe on his own. A break from the C1 to C3 vertebrae severs the nerves to the diaphragm and typically ties someone to a ventilator.

Don's injury high on his spinal column was similar in location to the injury suffered by the late actor Christopher Reeve. In 1995, Reeve broke his neck after being thrown from his horse during an equestrian event in Culpeper, Virginia. The wealthy actor and celebrity would go on to head an organization that raised millions for spinal cord injury research. Reeve was 43 at the time of his accident. He lived for nine years as a quadriplegic on a ventilator before dying at age 52 in 2004 from complications that reportedly stemmed from an infection caused by a bedsore.

4

Miracle Man?

At the time of his injury in 1987, Don was two months shy of his 25th birthday. He turned 60 on July 2, 2022. Don has spent more of his life immobile, than mobile. And he has far exceeded expectations for survival. The life expectancy for a ventilator-dependent quadriplegic injured at age 20, who survives the first year, is 17.1 years, according to the National Spinal Cord Injury Statistical Center. Survival decreases with age, with someone injured at age 40 expected to live 13.1 years.

"The problem with a C3 injury is that it impacts not only the muscles, but it impacts the respiration," said Ashraf Gorgey, director of spinal cord injury research at Central Virginia VA Health Care System (formerly known as the Hunter Holmes McGuire VA Medical Center) in Richmond. "It is a miraculous thing," he continues, referring to Don's longevity. "Usually, people don't make it that long on a ventilator."

A local colleague, Dr. William McKinley, director of

spinal cord injury medicine at Virginia Commonwealth University (VCU) Health System prefers the word "fortunate."

"He has beaten the expectations. He's definitely an outlier."

Susan Harkema, associate director of the Kentucky Spinal Cord Injury Research Center at the University of Louisville, considers Don's longevity "really unusual. I know a lot of people who have died at nine to 10 years."

Kemi Fakulujo, nurse manager for the spinal cord injury/complex care unit at Sheltering Arms Institute, a physical rehabilitation hospital in the Richmond region, agrees. "He's a very unique case," she said of Don. "It's not very often that you see someone with an injury at that high of a level live as long as he has."

Don's take on his survival is summed up with typical understatement: "It's not something I consider a remarkable achievement."

His humility belies the challenges of surviving a spinal cord injury. Patients like Don who stay on a ventilator are more susceptible to pressure ulcers, bladder and respiratory infections, and other life-threatening issues.

After dislocating his neck, it took Don months of speech therapy before he could speak again. Since his body no longer regulates autonomic functions such as body temperature, he goes outside only in temperate weather, giving him a small window in the summer and winter, or he will become too cold or overheated.

One of the biggest adjustments for quadriplegics is a lack of privacy. "When you need medical procedures every four hours and help with daily activities of living, you throw that out the window," said Don. Throw in possible problems that can arise from being hooked up to life support, and it's easy to see why Don requires 24-7 home health care.

Overall, losing one's mobility is a traumatic adjustment that tests everything: a person's will, identity, family relationships and place in the world.

Reeve said on the jacket of his biography, *Still Me*, that after playing Superman in the movies, fans used to ask him, "'What is a hero?'" His response? "A hero is someone who commits a courageous action without considering the consequences—a solider who crawls out of a foxhole to drag an injured buddy to safety."

After he became paralyzed from the neck down, Reeve said his definition changed. "I think a hero is an ordinary individual who finds the strength to persevere and endure in spite of overwhelming obstacles…"

While Don shies away from being called a hero, he is unquestionably a survivor. How did he beat the odds?

Don decided early on that bitterness would not be a healthy response to his injury. He will tell you that he is not angry at the world, at God, or his rugby teammates. Yes, it was a big match the day he was hurt. Emotions and testosterone ran high. But he doesn't believe anyone intentionally tried to hurt him. To this day, Don said he enjoys watching rugby on television.

The key to moving on after paralysis, Don said, is acceptance. Rather than ask "'Why me?'" the question for Don was, "'How can I move forward?'" That focus became a launchpad for recovery, as he journeyed from initial anxiety and depression over his limitations to a place of gratitude for the role he could still play. The process, though, didn't happen overnight. "It was a gradual process. It took me a while to come to terms with the disadvantages and the obstacles that were and are in front of me."

Don understands the dark valley traveled by many in the spinal cord injury community. "I understand where people are coming from," he says of quadriplegics who suffer from depression and suicidal thoughts. "They say, 'I don't want to live life this way.'"

At one point, early on, he felt the same way. Don's greatest fear was that he would live out his days in a nursing home. As time passed, and he learned ways to adapt, "It became more a matter of 'I don't want to quit.' Yes, it's been tough, but I'm still here. As long as I'm here, I'm going to try to make the best of it."

Don, like other quads, continues to hope for a brighter future. Since his injury, the field of spinal cord injury research has undergone a sea change, with assistive technologies getting better all the time. While scientists and researchers are yet to find a cure, they look to medical devices and experimental therapies to help patients stand, step, and, in some cases, walk with assistance.

Even without a medical miracle, Don's resilience has taken him a long way. Thirteen months after his injury, he returned to graduate school and finished a master's degree. He worked for a small business offering pre-design and assessment services for new construction and renovations. He got married and served as a stepfather to three children until the marriage ended in divorce. In many ways, he functions as a CEO of a small company, managing scores of home health-care workers over the years and battling government bureaucracy over disability benefits. He has held leadership positions in his church, the Church of Jesus Christ of Latter-Day Saints.

Helping Don along his journey is a supportive network. Family, friends, his church community, former rugby teammates and home caregivers have pitched in over the years with funding, care, and compassion.

Seeing Don navigate his challenges has had a profound impact on the way his friends see the world. "Being around a person with Don's injury, when you see other handicapped people, you have immediate sympathy and concern," said Chet Willis, a friend, and longtime trustee of the Help Don Succeed nonprofit trust fund. Recently when Willis was staying at a hotel, he spotted a young man in a wheelchair having dinner with his mother in the hotel's restaurant. "As they were leaving, I made eye contact, and I said something to him. They stopped, and we talked for about 30 minutes. I told him about my friend, Don, and how he's survived. Before I would have seen the guy, but I would never have talked with him."

For years, friend Steve Smith has driven Don to church on Sundays in Don's handicap-access van, a practice that stopped during COVID-19. A father of five, Smith has known Don for about 15 years. He noticed early on that Don doesn't complain about the devastating hand he was dealt. "I have never heard Don say, 'Poor me,' ever. He's never talked about his accident in a negative way, and I've known and talked with him a lot. That's what has made a huge difference in my life and in my family's life. If Don can be happy in his environment, then I can choose to be happy in mine ... Don is the friend who has changed my life, not because he's rich and powerful, but because he has persevered in the worst of circumstances, rising above paralysis to continue to make a contribution to his friends and community."

Seeing Don struggle with his physical limitations gives Smith a deep sense of gratitude for his own mobility. "I have left his apartment and not been able to drive away because of the tears in my eyes. It's beyond lucky, the freedom that you have. ... People see me helping Don, but people don't see how much he helps me. I'm really the lucky one."

Don takes such comments in stride. "Any time people say I'm special, the lyrics from the song "Electron Blue," by R.E.M., come to mind. 'And who am I? I'm just a guy, I've got a story like everyone.'"

"Everyone has trials and tribulations," said Don. "Everybody has obstacles to deal with."

Since becoming paralyzed, Don has experienced several

close calls. Once while being transferred from his bed to his wheelchair via a hydraulic lift, a caregiver accidentally dropped him, and he broke a leg.

Another time, his mother accidentally hit him while driving a renovated bread truck that served for a while as Don's handicap-access van. Unbeknownst to her, the truck had a loose gearshift. Don was in his wheelchair getting into position by the side of the van to board, when his mother started the vehicle. Instead of being in park, the van shot into reverse, and she ran into Don, knocking him and his wheelchair to the ground. Fortunately, he escaped without major injury.

Don has weathered urinary tract infections, a medical danger for quadriplegics, because they can lead to sepsis and a lethal blood infection. Don's latest brush with trauma came during the fall of 2021. After staying out of the hospital for years, he was admitted for what turned out to be septic shock. He spent several weeks at a hospital close to his home and then was taken to VCU Health System, (previously MCV), where his journey began more than three decades before.

During his six weeks of hospitalization, Don's lungs collapsed. He battled pneumonia, sepsis and, at one point, was put on a feeding tube. "When I saw him in the hospital, I didn't know if he was going to make it," said Angela Scharmer, a licensed practical nurse, who served as Don's lead home health nurse for 20 years. "They couldn't get his blood pressure under control. Everything was a mess."

Don survived what he jokingly refers to as his "holiday" and returned home shortly before Christmas. Since then, he has bounced back slowly. Don came home on oxygen, but has slowly been weaning himself off. "Dragging an oxygen tank around is a pain," he said.

Perhaps Don, rather than the beloved cats who share his apartment, is the one with nine lives. He scoffs at that notion, noting his survival may have more to do with a personality trait. "I'm pretty stubborn."

Part Two

Reset

5

Rehabilitation

After his spinal cord injury, Don stayed in the intensive care unit at MCV for nearly five months. The medical staff stabilized him, and doctors operated on his spine. Following the surgery, he developed a nasty infection in his neck, a complication that lengthened his stay. He remained in the ICU unit the entire time, Ellen said, "because that was the only area of the hospital with staff trained to care for patients on ventilators."

She and Don Sr. visited Don daily. In fact, Don had so many visitors—his girlfriend, mother, college roommate, fellow graduate students, rugby team friends, clergy—that Ellen said his room became known as "party central." He celebrated his 25th birthday at the hospital. "We were determined to do what we could to keep his spirits up. We even took his cat, Karl, to visit him, outdoors of course."

A complete injury to the spinal cord is like a sudden disconnect in the body's central nervous system. Nerves in the spinal cord transmit messages from the brain to the body and back again. After the injury to Don's C3 vertebra, damaged nerve fibers blocked the messages from the brain. That's why he lost sensation and movement below the level of his injury.

On September 22, 1987, Don was flown to what was then known as Shepherd Spinal Institute in Atlanta for rehabilitation. At that time, there were only three medical centers in the U.S. that offered rehabilitation to ventilator-dependent quadriplegics: Shepherd in Atlanta, Ga.; the Texas Institute of Rehabilitative Research in Houston, Texas; and The Craig Hospital in Denver, Colo. Today, there are 14 centers, not including programs offered at Veterans Administration hospitals.

Don's family opted for Shepherd in Atlanta because it was the first facility to have an available bed, and it was closest to Richmond. Plus, his father, stepmom, and members of Virginia's Medicaid office had toured the facility earlier. Don Sr. liked what he saw. "They were outstanding in terms of what they did with people."

Leaving family behind and going to Shepherd was hard on Don. Before the accident, "This was a time in my life that I was excited about. I had put in a lot of hard work at school and at work, and things were starting to come together. I was enjoying everything I was doing." He was especially excited about working with some professors on research projects, and he had a lead on a job in MCV's accounting department.

After his injury, feelings of anticipation and expectancy

were replaced with feelings of "sadness, disappointment, and frustration. Everything I had worked for to get to that point in my life, and now I was going to have to start over as best I could."

When he got to Shepherd, patients were required to undergo psychological testing. "This man kept asking me if I was angry. I said 'No, I'm not angry.' He said, 'At some point in the process of grieving, you're supposed to be angry.' He kept pushing this issue, and I finally said, 'Why? It's not going to get me anywhere.' I was thinking, 'What do I need to get back on track regarding my limitations?'"

The limitations were overwhelming. Don had to adapt in ways large and small. At his lowest point, he acknowledges there were times when he thought he would be better off dead.

Don's injury occurred during a sports event. Yet the leading cause of spinal cord injury in the U.S. is automobile accidents (38.2 percent), followed by falls (32.3 percent), and acts of violence, primarily gunshot wounds (14.3 percent). Sports/recreation activities represent another cause (7.8 percent), medical/surgical reasons (4.1 percent), and other (3.3 percent) according to the National Spinal Cord Injury Statistical Center at the University of Alabama in Birmingham, Alabama.

The U.S. sees nearly 18,000 new cases a year, which doesn't include people who die at the location of the incident causing the injury. About 78 percent of new spinal cord injury cases are male.

According to a 2013 study commissioned by the Christopher & Dana Reeve Foundation, an estimated 5.4 million people, or 1 in 50, live with some type of paralysis in the U.S. This includes spinal cord injuries, strokes, and people suffering with medical illnesses such as multiple sclerosis.

Facilities in Virginia provide care to nearly 3,000 people with spinal cord injury, according to Gorgey.

No matter the cause, coming to terms with a debilitating physical injury requires mental stamina. While a person may feel glad simply to be alive, it's difficult not to mourn what was lost. As the Shepherd staff worked with Don, showing him what could be done with adaptive technology, that support was like a beam of sunlight, burning away his doubts and depression.

One of the first things Don learned was how to get around in an electronic, sip-and-puff wheelchair. To go forward or backward, Don sipped air from a plastic straw attached to the chair or blew into it, the same way he operates his electronic wheelchair today. The chair weighs 400 pounds. Today's newer chairs are lighter and include hands-free technologies such as Bluetooth and smartphone apps to monitor activity.

Don learned to read with the help of an electronic page turner activated by a mouth straw, which seems antiquated today. Now he reads electronically on his computer through a Kindle application.

As part of occupational therapy, he learned to operate a computer. The interface Don left Shepherd with was a sip-and-puff Morse code activated through a mouth straw attached to his wheelchair. Back then commands were un-scrambled by what was considered a technological marvel at the time, a keyboard emulator. It translated the Morse code, allowing Don to send signals to the computer as if he were at a keyboard. Such systems are obsolete today thanks to voice recognition software.

Shepherd also trained family members in home care and health management. Since quadriplegics can't cough or sneeze, they are prone to respiratory infections, which increase the risk of pneumonia. To keep their lungs clear, they must be suctioned electronically several times a day. Home caregivers and family members also must change the position of quadriplegics while they are resting in bed—every four hours—or sitting in a wheelchair—every 90 minutes—to prevent bedsores.

Altogether, Don spent four months at Shepherd. During physical therapy, they tried to strengthen his neck and diaphragm muscles. Don could make small movements with his head, but he is unable to fully turn his head from side to side. No amount of exercising made him strong enough to get off the vent.

Another part of his rehabilitation involved outings to public places. The idea was to give wheelchair patients real-life experience in operating their chairs. Staff took him to the mall and the movies. There was a visit to former President Jimmy Carter's presidential library. Don's favorite trips? To sporting events like Atlanta Braves' baseball and Falcons' football games. While it was nice to get out, Don sums up rehabilitation like this: "It was a grind."

In the meantime, his father, stepmom, and mother were trying to figure out where Don would live when he returned to Richmond. Don had lived with his mother, Jutta Bridges, in Colonial Heights before his accident. He lived there while growing up and graduated from Colonial Heights High School. However, it didn't seem feasible for him to return since she worked full time, and her home was not handicap friendly.

"We visited a number of nursing care facilities," said Don Sr. He was troubled by what he saw. "The paralyzed residents didn't seem to have any quality of life. They didn't have their own phone or computer. They were kept alive and that was about it."

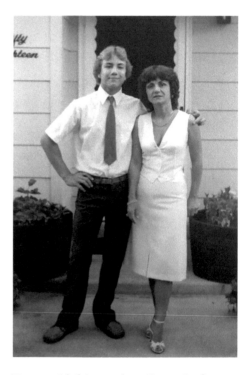

Had they selected a nursing home, Virginia's Medicaid plan would have paid for nearly all of Don's care. However, that wasn't the life Don Sr. wanted for his only son.

Don Sr., who was 45 at the time, and his

Don, with his mother, Jutta, in front of their home in Colonial Heights, Va., shortly before he graduated from Colonial Heights High School in June of 1980.

36-year-old wife began talking about caring for Don at home, against the advice of medical professionals. "I was determined that he wasn't going to a nursing home," said Don Sr. "They told me early on that most families abandon someone with that critical of an injury, and they put them in a nursing home, especially men."

Ellen doesn't remember how she and her husband arrived at the decision to let Don move in. They had been married for only a year and were still honeymooning when his accident occurred.

As the couple discussed the future for her husband's son, Ellen recognized these things:

• "I did not want to care for Donnie at home. I had a pretty good idea of how confining and stressful it would be. I never wanted children or had even babysat. I felt I was not cut out for it.

• "It would be wrong for me to put Don Sr. in the position of having to choose between me and our marriage or caring for his son.

• I loved Don Sr. and did not want to walk away and leave him to face this situation alone. It would be a shame to put someone of Donnie's age and intellect in a nursing home."

In the end the decision came down to this: "My love for my husband and having been raised to do the right thing."

Looking back, she finds it ironic that she would become Don's primary caregiver for seven years. "When Don Sr. and I were dating and things started to get serious, I thought to myself, 'Okay, Don has one grown son in graduate school who lives with his mother. I can deal with that.'

"You've heard the old Yiddish adage: 'Man plans, and God acts.' God obviously had a good laugh because He definitely had other plans for me."

6

Homecoming

G etting ready for Don's release from Shepherd in
January of 1988 provoked a flurry of activity for
Don's family. The Bridges sold Ellen's car and bought a van
with a raised roof to accommodate Don and his wheelchair.
They also sold the townhome they had just renovated, and
a rental home Don Sr. owned, so they could buy another
house with a basement that could be retrofitted for a person
with a spinal cord injury.

"We moved into the house in the fall of 1987 and had
only four months to design and build an apartment in the
lower level that included a kitchen and a bathroom with
a 6- by 8-foot shower that would accommodate a rolling
stretcher," said Ellen.

A team of volunteers, including Don Sr., Ellen's father, James Phlegar; and some of his retired friends did the
renovation and converted a garage into a living space for a
medical attendant since Don would need round-the-clock
help. "I wanted everything fixed up where he could be tak-

en care of very well," said Don Sr. "A lot of that planning came from what I saw at Shepherd and how they took care of Don there."

Don Sr. wanted the downstairs basement apartment to feel like home. He equipped it with a computer, Don's personal things, and a large aquarium for Don's exotic fish.

In the meantime, two of Don's classmates in the health administration graduate program at MCV, Stephens Mundy and Bill Jacobsen, started the Help Don Succeed (HDS) nonprofit public trust fund —a fund designed to help Don and other quadriplegics—and donations began coming in. A story in the local newspaper, the *Richmond Times-Dispatch*, raised awareness of Don's injury and preparations for his home care, prompting a response from some local businesses. Ellen said The Whitten Brothers car dealership in Chesterfield County offered the Bridges a good deal on a raised-roof van, because one of the younger Whittens knew Don. She was touched by offers of help from family, friends, and neighbors.

Before Don's release, Ellen, Don Sr., Sgueglia, and Don's friend and college roommate from Virginia Tech, Keith Fentress, went to Shepherd for training on spinal cord injuries and the accompanying physical challenges. "We learned about the ventilator, how to suction Don's lungs, catheterize his bladder and perform bowel programs," said Ellen.

Looking back, she adds, "I don't remember getting any counseling about the mental and emotional effects of spinal cord injury on the patient or caregivers, but that certainly should have been included."

While Don's home team was busy readying a place for Don to live, Don was trying to get his mind around the adjustments that come with being a quadriplegic. To go from life as an athletic young man who ran 20 miles a week to spending every moment in a bed or wheelchair is no small transition. While the wheelchair provided some freedom of movement, it also symbolized the loss of Don's mobility. In addition to a seatbelt, it came with straps that held his arms to the sides and leg straps to keep his feet securely moored in the foot pedals.

While at Shepherd, Don learned how to engage in daily activities. He also was encouraged to set goals. He wanted to finish his graduate degree and get some type of job.

Finally, the big day came. Don left Shepherd Spinal Center in late January of 1988 and flew back to Richmond. When his handicap-access van pulled into the driveway of his father's new home in the Brighton Green subdivision of Chesterfield County, he spotted a big sign that said, "Welcome home, Don."

Chet and Tammy Willis, neighbors who lived down the street, walked down the next day to say hello. "He was excited to be home," Tammy recalled. "His girlfriend was there. He was so handsome and so young."

Don was thrilled to be home. His new journey was beginning. While it was a scary new chapter, he told a local newspaper reporter a few weeks later, "I'm still here. There must be a reason. There are still a lot of things I want to do. I'm going to try and do them."

7

Starting Over

O nce Don settled into his new apartment, the hard
work began. Ellen became Don's primary caregiver. She was 11 years older than he. "I knew at the age
of 12 that I did not want children," she said. "So, to find
myself caring for a paralyzed young man, where I had to
catheterize him and intubate him was sort of a cosmic joke
on me."

Still, "I was glad to do it."

For the first year, Ellen split her time between hands-
on care for Don and matters related to his care. "I had to
find nurses who could sit with him to enable me to grocery
shop, to find sources for needed equipment not covered by
Medicaid, to investigate possible grants for which he would
be eligible and to raise money for his ongoing care from
civic and private groups."

Fundraisers included a fashion show held in conjunction with local churches and a Run for Don event held as

part of the Richmond Newspapers 26.2-mile Marathon.

When he was injured, Don was too old to be on his parents' health insurance policies. All he had was $25,000 in student medical insurance. That money was exhausted quickly as medical costs piled up.

After the accident, Don legally became a ward of the state. In Virginia, this designation qualified him for Medicaid benefits. The state's program paid for many expenses and some of his equipment. Today, a parents' income is not considered, and disabled people are not required to become state wards to receive state assistance.

Since Don wasn't living in a nursing home, state benefits would cover only a portion of his daily nursing care—six hours a day, five days a week. The aide assisted with basic activities such as dressing and bathing but was not trained to perform medical tasks. For in-home private nursing, the Bridges had to pay out of pocket, raise money or seek donations that were funneled into Don's trust fund, from which the nursing expenses were paid.

What the Bridges struggled to understand is that it would have cost the state more money if Don lived in a nursing home, where nursing care would have been covered. So why did regulations make it financially difficult to keep a loved one at home? They were saving the state money by caring for Don at home, but felt they were being penalized in the process.

Ellen spent the first year and a half with no live-in help, even though the Bridges had remodeled the apartment with that in mind. Instead, neighbors, family members, Fentress, and Don's girlfriend pitched in.

Since Sgueglia had taken the training, she served as Don's night nurse on the evening, 11 p.m. to 7 a.m. shift. She cooked for him, kept him company and got up with him during the night before leaving in the morning for a full-time job. She was 22 at the time. The two had been together a little more than two years.

It was a trying time in Sgueglia's life. Several months before Don's injury, her mother was diagnosed with brain cancer and underwent surgery and treatment. She was in re-mission by the time Don got hurt. The reoccurrence of her mother's cancer, inoperable the second time around, coin-cided with Don's return to Richmond from Shepherd.

Sgueglia lived with Don's family for a few months. Af-ter Don learned she had a fling with someone else, he asked her to leave. "He was understandably hurt," said Sgueglia. "I don't think he allowed himself to have the expectation that I would stay forever. Who knows what would have happened, but I had no plans to leave at that time. We looked into how couples with a disabled partner lived, had children, etc., while he was in the hospital."

Sgueglia was an important companion to Don at a time when his family had gone into survival mode. "We were in adventure mode," she said. "We were young. We wanted to go places, to do things." They would go out to dinner and the movies.

After their split, Sgueglia moved back to her parents'

home in Connecticut. A few months later, her mother died in September of 1988.

"It was hard on everyone, particularly Don, when she left," recalled Ellen.

Don was sad to see her go. The pretty Italian woman with long dark hair had been a source of support. It was comforting to have Sgueglia around, someone Don's age, who understood his difficulties in coping with a new life in ways his parents couldn't. She had been a big part of Don's life, cheering him on at rugby games and encouraging him in school.

When they fell in love and made plans to marry, Don was an able-bodied young man with plans of becoming a hospital administrator. As a quadriplegic, he still had plans. It was just going to take him awhile to figure it out.

Don wondered if he would find love again. Would anyone want him? Would he ever marry?

Those dreams seemed as deflated as a pair of old bicycle tires after Sgueglia left.

Her departure proved to be a double whammy. Unbeknownst to Sgueglia, while packing up her moving truck, Don's beloved cat of many years, Karl, jumped in. So the cat was gone, too.

What was hardest for Ellen with Don at home was the confinement. She spent most of her waking hours at home. Even after the family got live-in help, "Some people didn't stay long after we invested so much time and effort in training them. After a few months, they would leave with no notice. A lot of them stole from us or Donnie. It was constant stress, dealing with the state agencies and getting him what he needed."

Yet, she hung in there and got to know her stepson. Before the accident, Ellen had met Don only once at her and Don Sr.'s wedding reception.

Getting Don up and ready for the day was a laborious process that took nearly two hours. A typical day began at 7:30 a.m. That's when Don would wake and be fed breakfast in his hospital bed. After breakfast, Ellen donned sterile gloves to clean the tracheotomy at the base of Don's neck. Then she inserted a new inner canula in the tracheotomy to keep things as sterile as possible. When a cuff is let down on Don's tracheotomy tube, it allows air to pass over his vocal cords, so he can speak. Since he must wait for the ventilator to give him a breath, his speech is sometimes halting. But at least he can talk without a voice-assisted device.

By 8 a.m., the team would begin moving Don from his bed to a shower stretcher. The frame of the stretcher was placed on the bed while netting was placed under Don's body. It was tied to the stretcher in several places. With the help of a hydraulic lift designed and built by Don Sr., the aide raised the frame off the bed a few inches and placed it on the stretcher. Then Don was wheeled into the 6- by 8-foot, roll-in shower.

Using a spray nozzle, the aide washed Don's hair and the rest of his body, a luxury he remembers to this day. Few places he has lived since have had a shower large enough to accommodate his needs. Currently, Don settles for a bedside sponge bath.

"I didn't realize how good I had it at home," he said.

In the early days, Don would be disconnected from his ventilator during the shower, and Ellen would manually ventilate him using a small ambu bag. The small, handheld, self-inflating bag was used to force air into his lungs, so he could breathe.

After the shower, he returned to bed to be reconnected to his ventilator and dressed. The team employed the lift again to get Don into his wheelchair. Ellen brushed his teeth. Then, she inserted a tube into Don's tracheotomy tube and turned on a small electronic machine to suction Don's lungs. With quadriplegics, secretions tend to build up, so their lungs need to be suctioned several times daily.

On a good day, Don was ready to go by 9:30 a.m. He would spend the rest of the morning watching television or working on his computer. The simple sip-and-puff system that allowed him to operate the computer was a godsend in terms of communication. Plus, operating the computer gave him control over something in his life. He realized that his computer skills would be vital in terms of continuing with his studies.

After lunch, a physical therapist came to the house three times a week to exercise Don's muscles. On nice days,

he would roll his wheelchair outside and sit in the driveway. Sometimes friends came to visit. His good buddy
Fentress lived with the family for a year to help with Don's
care. His presence was therapeutic, said Ellen, because he
made Don laugh, cracking jokes about their time at school
and as fraternity brothers. Perhaps because he had known
Don before his injury, he didn't see him as disabled; he simply saw him as a friend. "I was determined that I was going
to do everything I could to help out with the situation,"
Fentress said.

Ellen also was touched by offers of help from neighbors who brought food or came to sit with Don so she
could run errands. "Tammy and Chet Willis, neighbors
who lived a few doors down, visited frequently, sat with
Don to relieve me, drove him places in his van, and threw
birthday parties for him."

Don's cheerful outlook lightened Ellen's load. "To this
day, I am in awe of Donnie's positive attitude and his refusal to feel sorry for himself. Those attributes, coupled with
his intelligence and wit, made caring for him easier than it
might have been otherwise. I learned that he is an extremely special and determined person. I also learned that I am
stronger than I realized."

By 6 p.m., Don Sr., who worked as a supervisor in the
purchasing department of the local utility company, arrived
home to lend a hand. He and Don would visit downstairs
while Ellen cooked dinner. Then the family would eat together. By 9:30 p.m., it was time for the couple to get Don
ready for bed. They suctioned him, catheterized his bladder,

and moved him from the wheelchair to the bed. Since the Bridges slept upstairs, they installed an alarm system to sound if Don's ventilator malfunctioned. On many nights, either Bridges or his wife would get up at least once to suction Don's lungs and to turn him to prevent bedsores. "I was up through the night a lot like with a sick child," Ellen recalled.

She has this advice for family caregivers: "Take care of yourself to the best of your ability. You can't provide good care for someone else if you are falling apart. Enlist as much help as you can from friends, family, community agencies. You will definitely need frequent breaks from your role as caregiver, and you may need financial help as well."

Despite the overwhelming obstacles of keeping Don at home, Don Sr. appreciated the time he spent with his son. The two had not lived together in years. Don Sr. had missed a few years of his son's life while serving overseas during the Vietnam War.

When Don left for college, Don Sr. and his first wife divorced after 22 years, and his son lived with his mother after that.

Don was born in Pisa, Italy, on July 2, 1962, while Don Sr. was stationed at a base near there during his Army career. He had been married to his first wife, Jutta, for two years before Don was born. He met Jutta earlier while he was stationed in Germany. After two years in Italy, the young family returned to the U.S. At that time, Don Sr. was assigned to the logistics unit at Fort Lee Army Base, just outside Petersburg, Virginia.

Don Sr. describes Don as "a very good kid. We used to hunt and fish together. He was good in school. He was prompt in everything he did. He couldn't stand a mess. He took good care of things. He didn't waste money." By the time Don was 12, he had his own bank account.

In high school, Don played recreational football in a local league. After graduating college, Don developed an interest in the health-care field after he began working at a local doctor's office in Colonial Heights. While attending graduate school at MCV in downtown Richmond, where Don Sr. worked at what was then Virginia Power after retiring from the Army, Don began seeing his dad again on a regular basis. "He would come down and eat lunch with me. That's how we got back together," said Don Sr.

That Don Sr. was now taking care of his son was a welcome change considering years of enmity between him and his ex-wife, a situation that made it difficult for Don to see his dad. When Don chose to live with him following his spinal cord injury, Sgueglia recalls, "His mother almost excommunicated him. But the father created a space where he could live independently."

The restoration of the father/son relationship was a balm to his son's soul, too, at a time when Don needed it most. In fact, he said the love and support he felt from his father, stepmother, and mother during the early years of his paralysis strengthened him for later years when he would be alone in terms of taking care of his needs.

8

Back To School

N ow that Don was settled in at home, he started
thinking about returning to school. He called his
professors at MCV who told him about a new master's
program in health administration. Don couldn't believe his
luck. All he needed was a computer, a modem, and a telephone to participate in what was the school's first electronic
classroom for graduate students.

The computerized instruction was designed for working professionals who wanted an advanced degree but
couldn't return to school full time. It was a perfect fit for
Don. Logistically, getting downtown every day for classes
while in a wheelchair and hooked to a ventilator would
have been difficult. "This was definitely the way to go."

Don signed on to the class of new-age learners. Little
did they know that the innovative program—the second of
its kind in the country back in 1988—would turn out to be
an early prototype for virtual learning.

Don began his studies in June of 1988. He would dial in to gain access to a computer conferencing system designed especially for MCV. The system provided directories where students could get assignments, confer with classmates, and review lecture notes from professors.

Don's computer link was his lifeline. "It felt good to be back at school and talking with other students." Besides the computer work, students were required to attend campus seminars five times over two years. The seminars, scheduled to last from six to 13 days, would be videotaped for Don. The cherry on top was that credits Don had completed towards his master's degree before his injury would be transferred to the new program.

Don graduated from Virginia Tech in 1984 with a bachelor of science degree in biology. He believed an advanced degree would help his employment opportunities. He dreamed of opening a group home for ventilator-dependent quadriplegics or finding a job in the health-care field.

Don thrived on the intellectual stimulation of an academic environment. He enjoyed hearing the perspectives of the other students, most of whom were already employed in health-care professions. Despite his enthusiasm for school, schoolwork itself proved to be a mountain of frustration. Back then, Don was operating his computer with a sip-and-puff Morse code. Using a mouth straw attached to his wheelchair, he gave commands by inhaling and exhaling.

Sip, sip, sip, sip, sip, puff. That's what it took to delete a single character.

It took Don three hours to compose a response to a single question. How would he ever graduate on time?

The state's Department of Aging and Rehabilitative Services came to the rescue with a laser head stick. The stick, held in place by a headband, enabled Don to point to letters on the computer that he wanted to strike, a faster method than sip and puff. Then the state equipped him with another improvement: the magic wand keyboard. The size of a postcard, it was mounted on a flexible arm attached to Don's wheelchair and electronically connected to his PC computer.

The magic wand computer had the same keys as a regular computer. By using a mouth stick, Don could touch

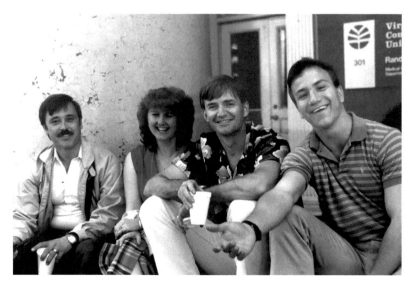

Don, far right, talking with some of his classmates in a graduate health administration program in Richmond in 1987 before he was injured playing rugby.

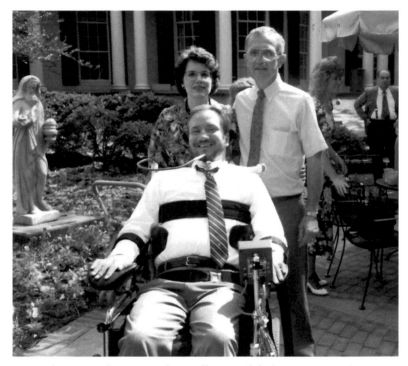

Don, shown with stepmother, Ellen, and father, Don Bridges Sr., during a reception for graduate students from the Medical College of Virginia on June 10, 1990.

the keyboard, and the strokes were electronically registered as keystrokes on the computer. On a good day, Don said he could type 20 to 25 words a minute.

What made Don happy was that he was moving forward and making progress. The rehabilitative services agency paid for his modem and the $2,126 fee charged annually under the executive study program. MCV waived the annual $2,540 tuition fee.

Time flew by. The next thing he knew Don was preparing for finals. Faculty assistants traveled to his home where he orally responded to test questions as opposed to taking written exams. Besides that adjustment, Don had the same requirements and deadlines for projects as other students.

On a clear summer's day, June 10, 1990, Don joked with classmates during a reception and graduation ceremony for master's degree recipients in the garden of the Valentine Museum in downtown Richmond. As the class of 21 students gathered for a picture, Don carefully moved his wheelchair into place. When his name was called, the class and those in attendance broke into hearty applause for the young man who showed such resolve in finishing his degree.

"For him to have achieved what he has achieved, I think it's an inspiration to other people," his mother, Jutta Jordan-Shahin (who had remarried) told a news reporter covering the graduation.

It was a proud day for Don and his parents. Unlike other graduates, though, Don had a unique concern: He couldn't make too much money on a job, or he would no longer be eligible for Medicaid, which helped pay for his medical supplies and some of his at-home nursing care, expenses that ran into thousands of dollars.

Unless he could strike it rich this would remain a lifelong concern, but Don didn't let it spoil the joy of the day. He thanked his family, friends, and the faculty and staff at MCV. "A lot of people have shown support and had a hand in this along the way."

9

Work

While Don was busy finishing up his graduate degree, his best friend Keith Fentress was lobbying on behalf of Don on Capitol Hill. The two had known each other since the fall of 1981 when they met at Virginia Tech while living in Pritchard dorm. Don was a sophomore and Fentress a freshman. When Fentress first saw Don, he noticed that he was wearing a shirt with a surfing motif. A surfer himself, Fentress asked Don if he surfed.

"He said, 'No.' And I said, 'You're a poser.' He said, 'You're an idiot freshman.' From that rocky start we became friends."

The two roomed together, pledged the same fraternity, Alpha Tau Omega, and played college rugby. They shared a love for the outdoors and frequently would get off campus to hike, fish, or ski, depending on the season.

In college, Fentress describes Don as driven. "I mean

this in a complimentary way because I wasn't. He was focused on a few goals, and he was driven to complete them.
There's no doubt in my mind that had he not had an injury
that he would be a hospital administrator of some large
hospital right now."

After he learned of Don's crushing injury, Fentress
said, "I was in focus mode. We've got to help him. What
training do I need to do? What law do I need to change?"

After Don returned home from the Shepherd rehabilitation program, Fentress was working part-time as an
intern for a health-care group in Washington, D.C., and
living with Don's family in Richmond the rest of the time
to help with Don's care. To make his case on Capitol Hill,
he wrote a paper based on a cost analysis comparison for
a ventilator-dependent quadriplegic living in a group home
with other quads versus living in a nursing home. "It was
cheaper for the government, and it was a better quality of
life," he said, all the while thinking what his friend might
do after he completed graduate school.

Fentress began to lobby legislators' offices to see if
there was interest in drafting a bill to support such homes.
One staffer asked him, 'How many of these people are
there in the U.S.? How many in my congressman's district?'
"That's when the bright lights flashed," said Fentress. "The
system isn't going to listen because there aren't enough
Dons out there."

Something good, though, came from his efforts.
"During my research, I ran into a woman who had several

group homes in California, and she said, 'If you get Don here, he can be an administrator at one of our homes.'"

Fentress told Don about the offer. "I tried. I pushed. But Don had so many things to worry about with his health and being close to his family [his main support system] that, at that time, leaving was terrifying."

After Don obtained his master's degree, Fentress hired him to work part-time for a small company he had started. Fentress Inc., which is still going today, offers pre-design and assessment services for new construction and renovation projects, with an expertise in courthouses.

Don's job involved the use of geographical information systems for mapping, work he could do on a computer from home. Fentress Inc. was based in Maryland, where Keith lived, and it had a couple of clients in Richmond. "We used to travel down to Richmond to hold meetings on a regular basis, and we would meet with him there, so he could be involved."

In June of 1990, Don served as a co-best man in Fentress' wedding. His family traveled to Maryland for the event, and Don dressed in a tuxedo like the other groomsmen. "I knew he couldn't do all of the requirements, so I had co-best men," said Fentress. "It was a great experience."

After two years of working for Fentress, Don was let go. "He had so many other distractions and priorities," said Fentress. "One of the hardest things I ever had to do was let him go."

While Don made inquiries into other computer-based jobs around Richmond, he learned quickly that most companies weren't looking to hire a ventilator-dependent quadriplegic. This was in the early days of the Americans with Disabilities Act (ADA), passed in 1990. Back then some employers weren't knowledgeable about the act's requirements, nor did they seem interested in making accommodations for a disabled person when they could hire an able-bodied person to do the work.

In 2021, the Virginia General Assembly passed a new law that expands disability protections. It added disability as a protected category under the state's existing Virginia Human Rights Act, requiring employers to provide reasonable accommodations to workers with disabilities. The law applies to employers with five or more employees, exceeding the requirements of the federal ADA, which applies to businesses with 15 or more employees.

When looking for employment, Don is restricted by income requirements. If he makes too much, he could lose a main source of income, Social Security disability insurance. In 2022 disabled people couldn't earn more than $1,350 per month ($2,260 for blind workers), if they wanted to remain eligible (not counting income from investments, spousal income, and other assets). That translates to $16,200 a year, only slightly above the federal poverty level of $13,350 for a single-person household.

Supplemental Security Income (SSI), another federal source of income for some disabled people, deducts 50 cents for every dollar earned over $85.

Beneficiaries of Social Security Disability and SSI can participate in federal work incentive programs, Ticket to Work and PASS (Plan to Achieve Self Support). They allow people to retain benefits for a time while training or exploring employment, including self-employment. Under Ticket to Work, people must work with approved employment networks that contract with the Social Security Administration. PASS requires a specific work goal within a reasonable time frame, and the job should allow someone to earn enough to reduce or eliminate their need for benefits. The SSI benefit may increase during employment training to help defray costs for training, tuition, supplies, and adaptive technology. The work plan must be approved by the Social Security Administration.

State Medicaid, including Virginia's program, also ties eligibility to income. This is the program that pays a good portion of Don's private home nursing care.

Unfortunately, working is a catch-22 for Don. If he makes too much, he will be penalized and lose his benefits. Yet trying to find a high-paying job to cover all his expenses is a challenge with his severe disability. Don would need an annual salary of more than $100,000 a year to pay for a portion of home nursing costs, prescriptions, and other living costs including electric, gas, and telephone service.

10

Spiritual Hunger

"*Hast thou not known? hast thou not heard, that the everlasting God, the Lord, the Creator of the ends of the earth, fainteth not, neither is weary? there is no searching of his understanding. He giveth power to the faint; and to them that have no might he increaseth strength. Even the youths shall faint and be weary, and the young men shall utterly fall: But they that wait upon the Lord shall renew their strength; they shall mount up with wings as eagles; they shall run, and not be weary; and they shall walk, and not faint.*"

Book of Isaiah: 40: 28-31 (KJV)

Eight years after injury, Don's life had settled into a routine. He oversaw his staffing, assisted with fundraising, visited friends and neighbors, and enjoyed outings to places like Dena's, his favorite Greek restaurant. Occasionally, he would attend fundraisers such as the annual golf tournament sponsored by the James River Rugby Club.

Life was okay. Friends his age were moving on. Many were married and starting families. He yearned to be part of a community. He noticed that one of his caregivers always spoke with enthusiasm about the church studies and social activities associated with his church, The Church of Jesus Christ of Latter-day Saints, more commonly known as the Mormon church. As a child, Don wasn't taken to church regularly, so he was curious about the man's religion. He had attended church "here and there," as a young adult, attending Mass occasionally with a former girlfriend and visiting the local Methodist church where his stepmother went. "I believed in God. I believed in Jesus Christ. But I wasn't spiritually mature."

Don's interest in religion "went all the way back to high school. It seems like I've always known someone who was a member of the church. I wasn't familiar with the gospel, but I always had a good impression of the people."

Don asked the caregiver to bring him a copy of the Book of Mormon, but the caregiver kept forgetting. One day, while watching television, Don saw an advertisement with an 800 number people could call if they were interested in getting a copy of the Book of Mormon. He called, or as Don puts it, "I invited myself."

Two days later, "Two young women showed up at the door." They were missionaries from the Mormon church. "I invited them in. We started talking, and I invited them back." Don continued his study with the missionaries, taking lessons in theology.

It wasn't long before Don began attending services with the missionaries. In the Mormon religion, congregations are organized by geography into wards, and each ward worships at a chapel. The chapel is led by a local bishop, a lay leader. A unique aspect of the Mormon church is that at the local level, it's strictly a lay ministry, with people giving their time and money to carry out the church's mission.

The more Don learned about the doctrines of the church, the hungrier he became for scriptural knowledge. He read the Book of Mormon from a CD on his computer, the Doctrine and Covenants, a collection of divine regulations given to prophet Joseph Smith and other church leaders for the establishment and regulation of the church; and the Pearl of Great Price, a selection of materials revealing significant aspects of the faith and doctrine of the Mormon church. He also read the Old and New Testaments of the Bible. After three months of attending worship at his local chapel, meeting members of the congregation and studying, Don decided to join.

For him, it was a momentous decision. At age 33, "I had finally matured to take on the covenants that we make with the Lord when we are baptized." Since Mormons require baptism by full immersion, the next step would prove to be tricky for Don because of his tracheotomy, the opening in his neck that allows for a tube to be placed into his windpipe, so air can enter his lungs, allowing him to talk.

Since Don had a trach and was connected to a ventilator, church friend Steve Smith said the local ward in Chesterfield County had to get permission for his baptism from the highest echelons of the church in Salt Lake City. "The baptism itself tells you how committed Don was," Smith said.

The special service for Don's baptism took place on Sept. 3, 1995. Before he was submersed briefly in a tank, Don said he and one of his caregivers figured out a way to stop the tracheotomy from filling with water. "We took an occlusive dressing that was waterproof and put that around the trach. Then we cut a piece of cork, like a wine cork, that fit right into the end of the trach. They put me on a wooden ambulance backboard, and then they lowered me down."

Was he scared? "No, I knew that Jesus was not going to let me drown for following his commandments," quips Don. He figures he was under the water for about a second, before being popped up. Still, the baptism made Don feel like a full-fledged member. On the day of his baptism, he was given a copy of the Book of Mormon signed by the bishop.

Everyone in the church's lay ministry is expected to contribute to the work of the church. Don has taught adult and youth Sunday school classes and served as superintendent of the Sunday school program.

The weekly church service on Sunday typically lasts for two hours. It begins with a sacramental meeting, where members are served the sacraments of bread and water. Then several speakers give a short speech. Don has been called upon to speak. "It's a wonderful opportunity for members of the congregation to be able to see this inspirational man share his thoughts of the gospel of Jesus Christ," said Aaron Gregory, bishop of the Brandermill Ward where Don attends.

The main meeting is followed by Sunday school. The local chapels, open to the public for worship, are not to be confused with Mormon temples, where special ceremonies, such as weddings take place. Typically, temples are not open to the public, except for a short time when a temple first opens.

Members drive Don to church, visit him at home for game nights and holidays and keep his fish tank cleaned. Don has recruited some of his nursing care through the congregation, and the church, at times, has pitched in funds to help pay for his nursing care.

"We do our best to assist Don as we are able," said Gregory, who is an attorney by profession. However, he adds, "It is not in Don's normal disposition to say, 'Help.' He is very independent."

Before Don returned home from a recent hospitalization, a group of women from the church cleaned his apartment thoroughly. "Everyone loves Don, and everyone wants to help him," said Gregory.

"The flip side is Don providing service to us. Don has a calling in our ward." His current job is ward communication specialist to the bishop. This involves sending out news and birthday greetings to members through email.

Having a spiritual home, says Don, gives him a purpose. "I've wondered for a long time, 'Why am I still here?' The reason I'm still here is to help others."

Don, who has very little family, adds that a supportive church community makes made him feel less alone in the world. "A lot of people in my situation end up isolated." When he wasn't attending church regularly during COVID-19, because of the risk of infection, he said, "I missed the fellowship. I missed taking the sacraments."

Don gives a portion of his income to the church, in what is known as tithing. He also strives to fulfill the mission of the Church of Jesus Christ of Latter-day Saints. "We believe we are here to learn as much as possible to become as Christ-like as possible."

Gregory said Don's presence motivates others. "I've heard it from so many people. You see Don with this obvious physical limitation and to see the kind, gentle and devoted soul that he is despite those circumstances, it helps put things in a very different perspective… Of course, he gets discouraged at times, but overall, you can tell he is at peace. He chooses to be at peace; he chooses to find joy in difficult circumstances. That's part of what inspires me and others to know Don. I feel like every time I meet with Don, I come away thinking very differently about what may be troubling me."

The bishop shared that he and his wife lost their fifth and youngest child when the baby was three months old. "That's been a hole in my heart and in my wife's heart the entire time, even though time helps to some degree. It's an example of a significant challenge in our life, which has nothing to do with the challenge that Don is facing, but to see how he deals with his circumstances and his challenges has been so inspirational to me in terms of dealing with the loss of a child."

One of the tenets of the Mormon faith is that after death members will have an opportunity to be resurrected and to a perfect body. "I think that is something that brings a lot of light and hope and peace for Don. Knowing that while he struggles with his current situation … he knows that isn't the end. There will come a time when he will be restored to a perfect body, that he will regain his strength and be able to move. I think that's an anchor for him," said Gregory.

Besides the promise of a new body in eternal life, the church also was the place where Don found something many men aspire to in this life: a wife.

11

Marriage, On His Own

I t isn't easy to meet a marriageable woman when a
young man lives at home with his parents. There was
someone, though, who sparked Don's interest at his local
Mormon church. Her name was Lori-Anna. At the time,
she was a divorcee with three children: two 12-year-old
twin boys, and an 8-year-old daughter.

At first, the romantic spark wasn't mutual. Lori-Anna
didn't seem interested. Then a writing assignment brought
the two together. Lori-Anna did some writing for a church
publication. In 1998, her assignment was to interview Don.
The interview went well. Don told her that he remembered
what she was wearing the first time he saw her: "A green
dress."

After a while, Don asked her out. They began spending
time together with her children at Don's parents' house.
Don liked Lori-Anna's children and wasn't intimidated by
the thought of a ready-made family.

A few months later, he proposed to her. She accepted. Don bought her a nice diamond ring. The wedding was set for April 30, 1999, in the Mormon temple in Montgomery County, Md. Since only church members are allowed in the temple, Don Sr. had to wait outside in Don's van.

Don Sr. opposed the marriage. "I tried to talk him out of it. I didn't think it would work out very well."

Lori-Anna said in a story published by the *Richmond Times-Dispatch* on June 18, 2000, that she met resistance from her family as well. "I had a lot of people in my family who dug their heels in. They thought it would be a burden for me. They pointed out the practical problems that would come up," she said. Later, she added, resistance turned to support.

The newspaper story celebrated Don's first Father's Day as a stepdad. He said he enjoyed having a family and being around children. He liked playing computer and board games, counseling the children about homework, hearing someone call him "daddy." "I've always wanted to be married and have children," he said in the story.

Following his marriage, he continued to live at home with his father for nine months while Lori-Anna's house was renovated to accommodate Don's medical needs and equipment. Ramps and decking were added to the exterior and interior so he could get around in his wheelchair. A bathroom was modified, and a hydraulic lift installed in his bedroom, so he could be transferred from his bed to his wheelchair. The home was set up so Don would live in the renovated basement but be able to come upstairs for family meals and activities via a ramp.

The renovation cost $55,200, said Willis, the largest single donation ever made to Don's trust fund. An anonymous group affiliated with Don's church in Utah picked up the tab. Finally, in February of 2000, the house was ready, and Don moved in. From the basement, he had a view of the backyard, where he could watch the children play.

At first things went well. The family ate dinner together. Don and Lori-Anna taught a children's Sunday school class. Don participated in the baptism of his stepdaughter by getting into the church's baptismal font once again, wheelchair and all, with help from some muscular church friends.

While he enjoyed the family aspects of marriage, there were problems and challenges as well, including Don's medical care. By the end of the year, the marriage crumbled. It's not a topic Don cares to discuss except to say, "I wasn't happy."

For the first time since his injury in 1987, Don was on his own. Don Sr. and Ellen had divorced in 1995. When Don moved to his wife's house, Don Sr. relocated to DeLand, Florida. Consequently, Don, 38, had no place to live. Then Laverne Lumzy, one of the home health nurses who helped care for Don while he was living with his wife, came to the rescue. She invited Don into her home and let him live there for six months. "I had no place to go. She was an unsung heroine, a real angel," Don said.

At the time, Lumzy was setting up a group home,

because she wanted to stay home and care for her disabled husband.

After six months, Don said a family from his church invited Don to live in their mother-in-law suite. Don relocated to the home of Jim Townes in Chesterfield County, where he lived for about two years. Then he moved to an apartment in Henrico County so he could be closer to his mother, Jutta Jordan-Shahin, who also lived there in the county. He missed being in Chesterfield, though, close to his church and friends. With help from his mom and a social services worker, Don found a three-bedroom apartment in Chesterfield where he has lived ever since. A Section 8 federal housing subsidy makes the apartment affordable.

For someone whose biggest fear was ending up in a nursing home, Don has enjoyed the stability of staying in one place for nearly two decades. Living on his own puts Don in control over his help and his schedule. Still, he admits, "Anxiety is an unwanted friend."

What if a home health-care nurse quits? What if the trust fund runs out of money? What if his ventilator breaks down in the middle of the night, and a nurse doesn't hear the alarm in time?

When life gets too stressful, "That's when I have to slow down. Instead of looking at the big picture, I take one little task at a time, so I don't get overwhelmed."

His apartment was not designed to be handicap accessible, but Don makes do. He is thankful to have a roof over his head and enough space to house his aquarium and his cats, who frequently snuggle with Don on the bed.

He can't feel the softness of their fur, but their purrs of contentment and displays of affection bring him joy. One of Don's cats, Albert, a beautiful orange tabby, lived to be 18. Losing Albert was like losing a best friend, said Don. Sometimes he swears he can see Albert, or at least a vision of him, walking around his bedroom, welcoming Don home.

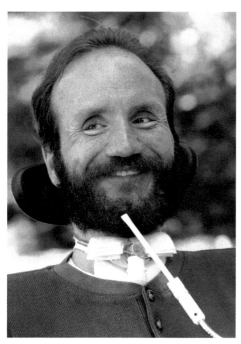

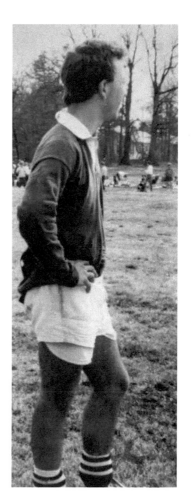

Top left: Don, at age 38 in 2000, shortly after his marriage. Photo courtesy *Richmond Times-Dispatch*.

Don (in top photo at right and in foreground of bottom photo) at a rugby team practice sometime in the early 1980s. Despite an injury during a game that dislocated his neck and left him paralyzed from the neck down, rugby remains one of Don's favorite sports.

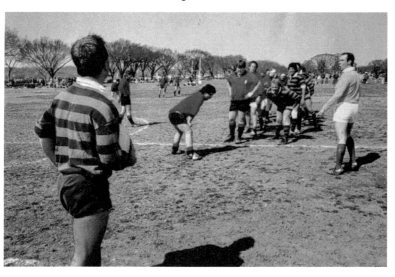

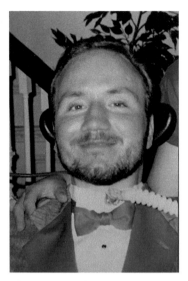

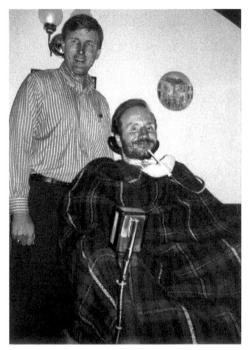

Above: Don decked out in a tuxedo and bow tie at the wedding of his friend, Keith Fentress, in June of 1990.

Don, relaxing at home with Chet Willis, frequently wears a blanket to stay warm.

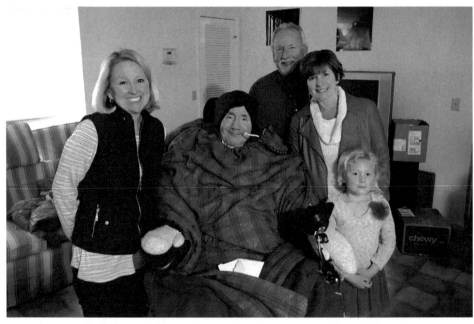

Don during a holiday visit in 2019 with Tammy Willis, (at left), her granddaughter, Grace Dean; and (at right) Paula Squires and her husband, Dean Squires.

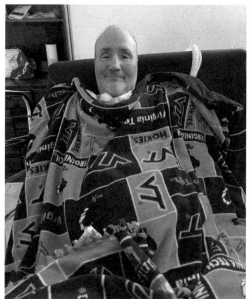
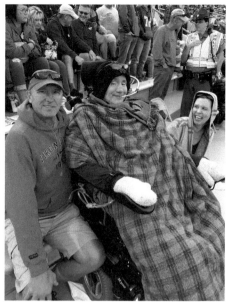

Above: School spirit—Don, who graduated from Virginia Tech in 1984, dons the school colors at home and while cheering at a football game in 2019. He's with Chet Willis, left, and caregiver, Neana Hines.

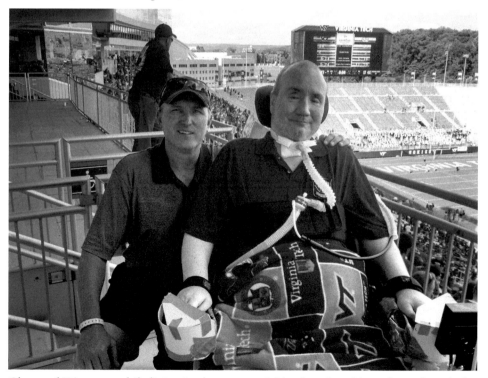

Chet and Don met while living in the same neighborhood and have been friends for 34 years.

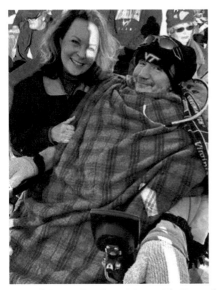
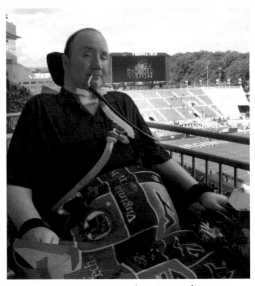

Friend Dana Ruder visits with Don during a game. He enjoys the view of Lane Stadium.

Below: Don looks forward to "game day," his annual outing to a Hokies' home football game. Chet Willis, a fellow Virginia Tech alumnus, drives him to Blacksburg where Don watches the game along with thousands of other fans. "Sitting in Lane Stadium with 65,000 people is a breathtaking thing," says Don.

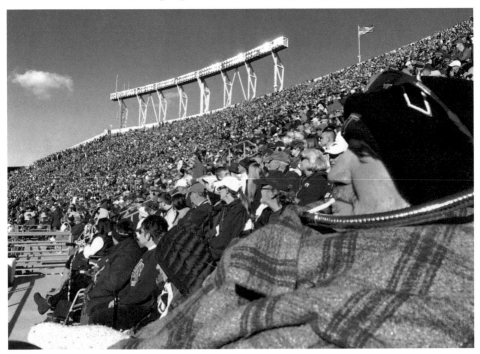

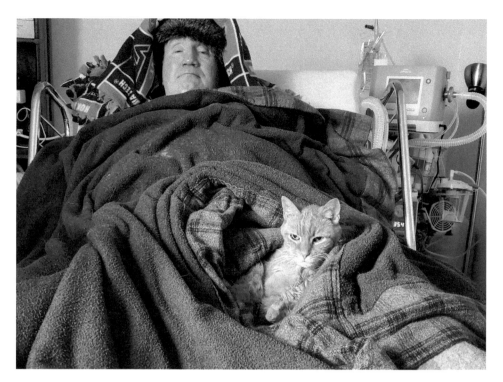

Top: Don's cat Albert could frequently be found lounging in Don's bed. Bottom: Angela Scharmer worked with Don as a home health nurse for 20 years. She retired in 2022 and frequently stops by to visit.

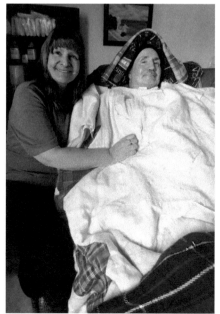
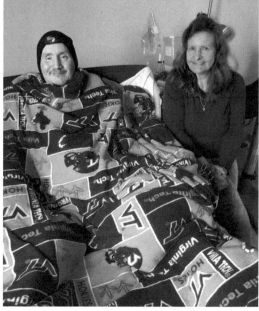

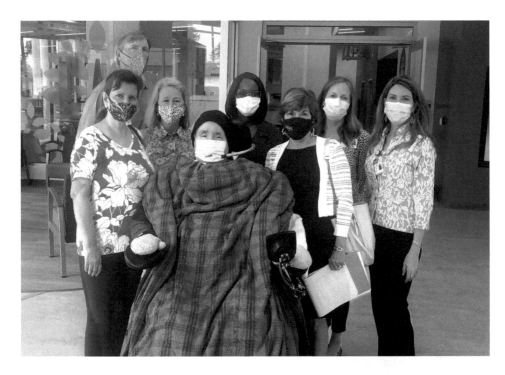

Above: Don is masked and ready for a tour of Sheltering Arms Institute, a physical rehabilitation hospital in Goochland County, Virginia. Accompanying him on the tour in May of 2021 were (from left front row) nurse Angela Scharmer and author Paula C. Squires. On back row (from left) are friends Chet and Tammy Willis and members of the hospital's staff, Kemi Fakulujo, Joanna Moore, and Stephanie Sulmer. Photo courtesy Sheltering Arms Institute.

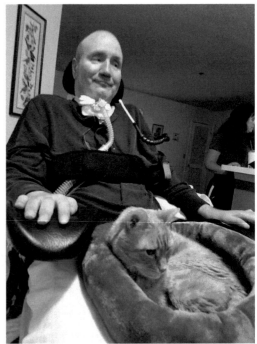

Albert served as Don's loyal companion for 18 years before he died in 2021.

Part Three

The Help

12

Angels and Devils

O ne of the greatest challenges for quadriplegics
living at home is finding dependable caregivers.
Over the past 35 years, Don estimates he has hired more
than 100 people, from licensed practical nurses to personal
care assistants. It's a merry-go-round, with people jumping
on and off the staffing schedule that is Don's life. Keeping
track of the personnel, their schedules and payments takes a
lot of Don's time.

Some workers stay for years while others barely last
a day. The COVID-19 pandemic has made staffing more
difficult, with health-care workers leaving the profession,
reducing the worker pool. Plus, in Virginia, there is a short-
age of private duty nurses because rates paid by Medicaid
for nurses serving disabled people—$34 to $38 per hour—
are lower than the $60-to $65-per hour nurses can earn
from private insurance companies.

Don's stories about the help reveal the best and worst
in human behavior. "Most people are really good," he said.

However, the colorful cast of characters who have passed through his life come in all stripes. Some have failed to show up for work while others have stolen from him.

Items gone missing through the years include CDs, DVDs, jewelry, and medication. One male worker charged 800 calls to Don's cell phone while another assistant took his handicap-access van for a joyride without permission. It was found later, abandoned, in a part of Richmond known for drug dealing. Some of his female aides have behaved unethically as well. "I've had unwanted advances from three women," said Don.

His most harrowing experience occurred when a new caregiver failed to hear the alarm going off on his ventilator. Don was sitting in his wheelchair in his bedroom. The caregiver was in the living room, a short distance down the hall. Since the ventilator had shut off and Don couldn't speak, "I started making this kissing sound," he recalled, the same sound he uses to call his cats.

The caregiver thought he was calling his cats and didn't respond. Meanwhile, "I'm starting to get light-headed from not being able to breathe. The last thing I heard before I passed out was, 'Why is the ventilator alarm going off?' The next thing I knew there was an ambulance, and they were bagging me with an ambu bag."

Don was taken to the hospital. When he returned home, he said paddles from a heart defibrillator were still attached to his chest. "She quit right then," he said of the new aide.

Don staffs for three shifts: 7 a.m. to 3 p.m., 3 p.m. to 11 p.m. and 11 p.m. to 7 am. Since he is paralyzed, Don is eligible for the state's Coordinated Care Plus Medicaid Waiver, a program that provides services to disabled people in the community. In Don's case, the waiver pays for two eight-hour nursing shifts a day, seven days a week, including equipment, supplies and anything that is medically necessary. That's a big improvement from the one six-hour shift per day during the week that was authorized when Don was first injured.

Nurses perform medical tasks, such as suctioning, cleaning Don's tracheostomy and monitoring his ventilator. According to Rebecca Stricklin, a care management specialist with the Virginia Department of Medical Assistance Services, which administers the waiver program, there are nearly 300 people in the state receiving benefits who are ventilator-dependent quadriplegics. About two-thirds of them are children, she added, who suffer from birth defects.

With good help hard to find, Don doesn't always have two nurses on staff. In the past, he has gotten by with a nurse working the early shift and personal care assistants working the other two shifts. To help in recruiting, he recently bumped his starting wage for an aide. Angela Scharmer, a licensed practical nurse who headed Don's home care for 20 years until she retired in February of 2022, earned about $40,000 a year. All told, the trust fund picks up about $75,000 a year in nursing expenses not covered by the state, said Willis.

Scharmer, 65, began working for Don in 2002. While she could have earned more in a private facility, that's not her calling. "When you work in a facility, you don't have the same one-on-one with a client. You're busy charting, passing meds, talking with the family, answering the phone. With Don, it's more like old-school nursing where you can spend time with the patient."

As the most senior member on his staff for two decades, Scharmer served as the glue who held the operation together. If someone didn't show up because of illness or bad weather, she worked a double shift. She bought most of Don's groceries and made sure he received flu and COVID-19 shots.

Another important task was teaching other home health workers how to operate the ventilators attached to Don's bed and his wheelchair. Today's digital ventilators can be preset and aren't hard to monitor, said Scharmer. However, when someone is on life support, staff needs to know how to troubleshoot if the alarm goes off. Today, Don's vent pumps 12 to 14 breaths into his lungs per minute. When Don speaks, the vent automatically adjusts to give him more breaths.

Born in Glasgow, Scotland, Scharmer speaks with the lilting accent of her native country. She has known Don for so long that she describes their relationship as that of a brother and sister. Don jokingly referred to her as "the evil, older sister," because she cracked the whip when it came to organization. "He may not be in a facility, but we ran it like a facility in that it makes more sense and keeps everything more organized," said Scharmer.

That means the staff does the same thing—bathing, eating, medical checks—at the same time on most days. Don calls it his "Groundhog Day." When he goes to see the doctor or, better yet, travels to a Virginia Tech football game, he enjoys the escape of his "groundhog" routine.

Kidding aside, he respects Scharmer and the devotion she showed to her job. When she was on duty, the two would laugh and joke together. "We're not alike at all in nature," said Scharmer. "I do everything fast; he does everything slow. He's an old soul; I'm a young soul. We are completely opposite. I've wanted to be something in his life that was constant. When you don't have [much] family, you have to have someone to trust and someone who has your best interests at heart."

"She's very thoughtful," Don said of Scharmer. "She cares about me, or she wouldn't have stayed around so long. She could have been making a lot more money elsewhere."

On holidays like Easter, Thanksgiving and Christmas, Scharmer invites Don to her home. "He's like a member of the family. Just another potato in the pot. We open our presents together. I open his for him. He's comfortable here. He'll sit at the table with me. I'll feed him. Everyone will be talking. It's just like a normal thing."

Despite her mother-hen tendencies, Scharmer encouraged Don to live as independently as possible. "He can use a computer, and he can use a telephone. So, when we needed another nurse, I would tell him, 'You make the calls.'" Don finds help through staffing agencies, newspaper advertisements and personal referrals.

Scharmer's journey with Don has taught her many lessons. "I've learned not to complain about the small things in life. Somebody always has it worse. Things that used to bother me don't bother me now. You realize how blessed you are."

She realized early on that it was important to see Don beyond his disability. "People like him don't want to be treated differently. They don't want to be treated like some fragile flower, like you're sorry for him. Don wants to be treated like a regular guy."

Scharmer's No. 1 rule for home health nurses tending a paralyzed client: "Don't take everything personally. They're going to have days where they probably hate the world and that's understandable ... You can't take that home with you or it will interfere with your life. You have to be able to switch that off."

A few weeks before her departure, Don joked that he already was experiencing "separation anxiety." No need to worry, responded Scharmer. "I'm just a phone call away. If anything goes down, I want them to call me ... I'm not abandoning him; I just don't want to be on a schedule anymore."

She expects Don will be fine because of his resilience. "He's like a phoenix rising from the ashes ... It's almost like every time something happened, God sent him an angel."

Another compassionate assistant to Don was Bill Lockwood. He worked for Don for 14 years before retiring. Lockwood, who served in the Virginia National Guard, was well-read, and the two enjoyed discussing philosophy, history, and religion. "He was good for Don," said Scharmer, "a male, a great and caring person with similar interests. They would always joke around."

Neana Hines, a certified nurse's aide, worked with Don for five years. She left in January of 2022 after serving as Don's "personal assistant, primary cook, cleaner." Hines said Don's greatest strength as a people manager was his "patience. That man has more patience with new assistants. He saw potential in me. He trained me. He never belittled my intelligence. He never made me feel small or stupid because I didn't get something right the first time. He's one of the best teachers I've ever seen. He should have been a college professor or a dean of a college."

Over the years Don has learned the key to managing caregivers. "It's about developing a good rapport and being appreciative of the help, showing and telling them that."

He's met people from all walks of life and developed friendships with some of his caregivers. In some ways, they are his eyes to the world since Don's ability to get out was greatly reduced during the pandemic. Entrusting your life to strangers is never easy, but it comes with the territory.

13

The Power of Community

"The greatness of a community is most accurately measured by the compassionate actions of its members."

Coretta Scott King

octors will tell you that a person's ability to thrive is largely influenced by two factors: personal motivation and a good support system. Over the years, Don has been blessed with a strong network of support from family, friends, neighbors, his church, his former rugby club, and even total strangers.

Upon learning of Don's struggle to acquire a newer model handicap-accessible van, the late Doris Buffett, a philanthropist, and sister of billionaire investor Warren Buffett, donated $25,000. Ms. Buffett headed the Sunshine Lady Foundation, a private family foundation that used her investment funds and a stock gift from her famous brother to help people in crisis.

In a letter to Ms. Buffett explaining his situation, Don wrote, "I cannot breathe on my own, but the accident didn't injure my brain. So, I have tried to continue on life's journey, getting a master's degree and living independently as best I could."

Ms. Buffett was glad to be of assistance. In a note to the journalist who brought Don to her attention, she said, "Don is an amazing man. How many of us could handle his situation? Not me."

The bulk of Don's support comes from the local community. Many of the people who first assisted him when he was injured are still part of his life today. Others have drifted away. The ones who continue to give their time, talents, and money to help Don remain independent provide a powerful example of the good that comes from a collective effort.

One of the most faithful and generous contributors to Don's trust fund is a group called the James River Old Boys (men who played for James River Rugby Club during the 1970s and 1980s). It gives $1,300 a month, according to the club's historian Terry Byrd. Altogether, the group has donated more money to the HDS fund, $192,700, than any other entity.

To raise money, the club holds various fundraisers, including an annual golf tournament. It typically raises $6,000 to $8,000, although the tournament was canceled the two years of the pandemic. Fundraiser money goes into an account that is invested, with the group donating monthly to Don's trust. Byrd said the club's funds also have been used to pay college expenses for two children of a rugby player who died of leukemia.

"Our game plan was to raise enough money to put Bubba's kids through college and to help Don out." The children have graduated, and both played for the rugby club for a time, said Byrd. "Our money will run out eventually."

Byrd, who played with Don during his time on the team, said the club wanted to help him from the beginning. "I'm just amazed that he has done so well. I'm not sure I could do what he has done."

Another large donation, $25,000 in unrestricted general fund money, came from Don Sr.

Since Don's injury in 1987, the trust fund—founded with the mission to help Don and other quadriplegics live independently in the community—has generated $1.2 million in donations and earned $4,500 in interest, said Chet Willis, the fund's co-trustee. From that money, $1.1 million has been spent to help Don. Another $87,000 went to three other people with spinal cord injuries: a young man injured in a car wreck in 1992, a man who severed his spinal cord while diving into a pool in 2009, and more recently a man and former college buddy of Don's who suffered a severe stroke.

A total of 56 nurses and home health aides have been paid with monies from the fund. With money always going out for expenses, there have been times when the fund has nearly run dry. "There have been months when we have wrung our hands, and we [meaning he and his wife] have made up the difference. But somehow the money always comes in," said Willis.

Fentress and Ellen, who live out of state, are regular contributors. When Ellen and Sgueglia come to Richmond to visit friends or relatives, they go by and visit Don. While sometimes years slip by before she sees him, Sgueglia said, "We're still connected in our hearts."

Community groups have also pitched in. In the early days after Don's injury, two local churches in Chesterfield County, Bon Air United Methodist and St. Michael's Episcopal, sponsored a fashion show and other events with proceeds donated to Don's fund. In 1989, a "Run for Don" fundraiser tied to the local newspaper's annual 26.2-mile marathon, prompted pledges that raised $7,500. Groups like the Brandermill Rotary Club have contributed.

These gestures let Don know others care about him. It fuels his endurance and his hope.

While the trust fund serves as his pipeline to independent living, men and women do not live by bread alone. The Willis family has stood by Don's side from the beginning. Tammy and Chet Willis first met Don when they lived a few doors down from Don Sr.'s home in the Brighton Green subdivision in Chesterfield County.

Willis, four years older than Don, was a Virginia Tech alumnus like Don and a fellow Hokie football fan. "He loved football. We had this instant connection," said Willis.

Willis also worked as an engineer at the same utility company, now known as Dominion, where Don Sr. worked. He had heard about Don's injury through an employee newsletter. When Don returned to Richmond following his rehabilitation stint at Shepherd, "We got involved right away," said Tammy.

At first, Tammy would sit with Don so Ellen could run errands. Then Ellen trained Tammy on how to operate an ambu bag. Once a week, Tammy helped put Don to bed. "It took two people to get him from the chair to the bed. You would disconnect him from the ventilator and use the ambu bag to do the breathing for him to get him to the bed."

The family treated Don like a friend. "He would come to our house and have dinner," recalls Tammy. "We had no front stoop. He would come down in his wheelchair. The kids would sit on his lap, slide down his leg, put barrettes in his hair. Being an only child and not being around a lot of kids, he seemed to like it."

Willis was asked if he could help by writing checks from the fund to pay for Don's home nursing care. He became a fund trustee in 1989, a position he has held ever since. He assumed the responsibility, he said, because "This is something I can do… He'd become a real good friend, and you just do these things for friends."

Willis also is the person behind Don's annual trip to a Virginia Tech football game, an adventure Don looks forward to all year. Willis gets game tickets and drives Don three hours down Interstate 81 to Blacksburg in Don's van. A medical attendant comes along and usually a church friend, too. "Sitting in Lane Stadium with 65,000 people is a breathtaking thing," said Don.

The group sits in the handicapped area near the end zone where Don has a good view of the field and overhead jumbotron. Don enjoys seeing how the campus has changed since he was a student. "The growth takes you back a bit," he said, referring not only to expansions on Tech's campus, but Blacksburg's overall retail growth.

Decked out in game-day regalia—an orange and burgundy Hokie blanket and scarf and hat with VT insignia—it's easy for Don to wax nostalgic about his student days when he lived at Pritchard dormitory and dined at Dietrick Dining Hall or Squires Student Union.

What does he remember most? "Just the freedom of being on my own and doing what I wanted to do. Just being with friends."

Since it's a day-long event, everyone brings lunch to avoid standing in long lines to get fed. Willis picks a game, usually in late September or early October, when the weather isn't too hot or too cold. Overall, it's a fun fan day that fell by the wayside during COVID-19. Since he's on a ventilator, Don has avoided large crowds where the chance of infection is greater. He's counting the days to when he can rejoin the boisterous fans at Lane Stadium.

The Willis' say their friendship with Don has been life changing. "I've learned that you can overcome," said Tammy. "That there's nothing in life, with God's help, that you can't overcome, that you can't live with."

Willis has pondered on Don's life and his resilience. Not being able to move is a physical tragedy, notes Willis, an avid golfer. Being around Don makes him appreciate his own freedom of movement.

The Willis' believe one of the reasons Don has lived so long can be traced back to the tremendous amount of effort his father and stepmother put into keeping Don at home. Altogether, Don Sr. helped take care of Don for 12 years until his son married. "His dad's actions, the energy he poured into keeping him alive, set an example for him," Tammy said.

Tammy and Chet host Don Sr. when he comes from Florida to visit Don. Don feels lucky to have such caring friends. In a sense, they've grown up together, sharing in each other's lives for more than 30 years. If he needs help, Don knows he can call Willis. "Chet is honest and dependable. I can always count on him for a timely response."

Another constant in Don's life is his family doctor. Dr. Kevin Keller—the same doctor he used to work for and the one who rushed to the hospital the day of his injury— has served as Don's primary physician for more than three decades.

Typically, Keller sees Don twice a year unless a medical problem arises. Besides ensuring Don is up to date on vaccinations, Keller checks his overall health and looks for signs of respiratory infection and skin changes. Breakdowns in the skin are a common hazard for quadriplegics, because of their inability to change positions. To guard against bedsores, Don sleeps on a mattress that regulates air pressure.

When he first began treating Don, Keller said he sent letters to Medicare, successfully lobbying the federal agency to pay for sterile catheters. They guard against urinary tract infections, another enemy of quadriplegics. Don's catheter, which captures urine, needs to be removed three times a day.

That Don has remained healthy for so long is a feat Dr. Keller attributes primarily to Don and the good nursing care he has received at home. "Don is a big reason why he has stayed so healthy. He has taken charge of his health," said Keller, meaning both physically and mentally.

In all the years he has seen him, "maybe only once or twice can I remember Donnie feeling blue. He is not a woe-is-me kind of guy." In fact, Dr. Keller wishes he had more patients like Don. "I think about Don when I get a call from a patient who starts taking antibiotics one day and then calls the next day to question why they're not working yet. Here's Donnie on a ventilator for 35 years. How come he never calls? He's the gold standard."

It isn't just Don's attitude or injury that makes him special, adds Keller. At the time of Don's injury, "He was a single sibling on the verge of getting married. He had two parents who helped him in the beginning, but they're not in the picture now. His Mom [lives in a nursing home] and his dad has lived in Florida for years. He doesn't have a family. It's quite remarkable, beyond the injury, what he has been able to do for himself."

The two men share a love of fishing, and sometimes they talk about that as opposed to medical stuff. Once when Keller took a fishing trip to the Amazon River, he sent Don photos of some of the fish that were caught. Don knew the names of all the fish, he said. Dr. Keller never dreamed when Don first walked into his medical practice all those years ago looking for a job that the two would embark on such a long journey. "He's been inspirational and a tremendous help. We're joined at the hip."

Church friends provide another important network. From cleaning his van and fish tank to getting him to church, they spend time with Don on a regular basis. Friends provide the social interaction Don needs to stay positive. They affirm that he is more than his disability. Don is a son, a friend, an ardent Hokies football fan, a disciple of Jesus Christ and a tough guy to beat at board games.

Steve Smith should know. He plays Ten Days in Europe with Don, a travel game where players plan trips across Europe by land, air, and sea. "We're pretty evenly matched," said Smith. Yet occasionally Don outplays him with a strategic move.

Smith, who works in IT, wants to update some of Don's electronic accessories. "There's still work to be done," he said, "but doing the work with Don—notice I said with and not for— is fun."

The power of networking also extends to the spinal cord injured community. It has produced powerful role models, from the Paralympics to Hollywood's Christopher Reeve and academia's Brooke Ellison. Their success stories prove there is life beyond injury.

Brooke Ellison was paralyzed from the neck down at age 11 after being hit by a car. Ten years later, she graduated from Harvard University.

Her mother served as her roommate for four years to allay the school's concern about Brooke's need for 24-7 nursing care since, like Don, she breathes with a ventilator. When she spoke during commencement at her Senior Class Day, Ellison was on the brink of graduating with honors from one of the most prestigious schools in the country. "Miracles happen," she told her classmates. "They have happened to me, and they are happening to you. You need only look at the people in your lives in order to see them."

Ellison wrote a book about her time at Harvard, *Miracles Happen, One Mother, One Daughter, One Journey*, that was adapted into a television movie by Reeve. After earning her undergraduate degree in cognitive neuroscience, she went on to earn a master's degree in public policy from Harvard and a doctorate in sociology from Stony Brook University, where she is an associate professor of health policy and medical ethics.

Ellison speaks and advocates for people with disabilities at events around the country. During the COVID-19 pandemic, after she survived a bedsore that threatened her life, Ellison wrote a second book, *Look Both Ways*, that shares lessons learned after being paralyzed for 30 years. Like Don, she is a longtime survivor with a few bumps and bruises, but her can-do spirit and desire to give back haven't wavered.

14

Ripple Effect: How an SCI Affects Family and Friends

W hen someone is suddenly paralyzed, that person experiences a range of emotions, and so do the people around them: shock, grief, anger, fear, denial, loss, confusion.

Especially for families there is a ripple effect as they watch a loved one adjust to a disastrous turn of events. Family members and friends also may face changes if they assume a caregiving role. There are many resources, therapies, and treatment programs today to help people move on and lead productive lives. In the best-case scenario, the paralyzed person moves from helplessness to hope, boosting everyone in their inner circle.

Yet no matter how someone responds to their paralysis, it affects people around them in different ways, even years after the event. When asked what impact Don's injury had on their lives, some of the people closest to him spoke of loss and an inability to trust in the future. Others, seeing

Don rise to the challenge of living a new way, felt inspired and began to view the world with more appreciative eyes.

Here are their thoughts:

Donald Bridges Sr., Don's father: After Don Sr. and his second wife, Ellen, cared for Don in their home for nearly seven years, the marriage crumbled. Ellen served as Don's main caregiver. The couple worked as a team, ensuring that Don had what he needed. It was difficult, though, for the two of them to get time away since Don required 24-7 nursing care, and sometimes the help didn't show up. Don Sr., an alcoholic who had foregone drinking when he first married Ellen, began drinking again. "I got to drinking worse and worse and went up to the treatment center for a while."

He says his alcoholism started long before Don's injury. "I was an alcoholic before he got hurt, and then I started drinking more." He's been sober since rehab. Looking back Don said, "Ellen was a hero. She was an extremely good person. All I can do is admire her and thank her for everything she's done."

After Don Jr. married in 1999, nearly 12 years after his father moved Don into his home, Don Sr. relocated to DeLand, Florida. He found work at the local airport, helping to maintain planes used for the airport's skydiving training center. Don Sr. decided to try it and jumped 200 times. Even with Don Jr.'s history, "I never worried about getting injured," he said. "You're taking a chance on anything you do."

When his son was first injured, Don Sr. coped by helping to care for Don. "Now the only way of dealing with it
is staying away from him. It takes a toll on you. It hurts. I
come up and see him now, and it hurts. You would think
that would go away, but it doesn't go away."

Don Sr. flew to Richmond twice during his son's recent
hospitalization. He's on his second pacemaker and will
soon celebrate his 80th birthday. Had Don not married,
Don Sr. says he would have stayed in Chesterfield, providing a home for his son. "I would still be there with him. But
by getting out, he learned to take care of himself."

**Jutta Jordan-Shahin, Don's mother and Don Sr.'s first
wife:** Shahin resides in a nursing home and could not be
interviewed. Like other people dealing with aging parents,
Don worries about his mother and deals with the attendant
medical and legal issues.

**Ellen Eggerding, Don's former stepmother and Don
Sr.'s second wife:** Eggerding agrees that caring for Don put
pressure on the marriage. "Don Sr. and I had just been
married a year. If you're in a marriage or a relationship,
you have to nurture that. You've got to set aside couple
time. We couldn't do that. We were on duty on the weekends when the live-in help was off."

Yet something beautiful flowed from the arrange-
ment; namely, the rekindling of the father/son relationship.
"There was so much enmity between Don's mother and father, that he [Don Jr.] would try to keep the peace. Before,
he wouldn't let his mother know he was going to see his

father." Once Don Sr. and his son shared the same address, Don was no longer in the middle.

Don Sr. and Ellen divorced in 1995. Since then, Ellen has remarried. She lives in North Carolina and has taken up watercolor painting. Some of her waterfowl portraits hang in Don's apartment.

Patty Sgueglia, Don's former girlfriend: Don's injury in combination with the death of Sgueglia's mother shortly thereafter from cancer were pivotal events that affected her sense of permanence. "I've had no children, no long relationships and many residences."

Sgueglia said her priorities also changed. "When you have big things happen, you don't sweat the small stuff."

Now a resident of Florida, Sgueglia works in the insurance industry and recently visited Don during a trip to Richmond. "The single greatest testament to Don's courage and perseverance is getting through the day. Each day brings unexpected challenges and obstacles, which must be met ... It is astounding to witness Don's absolute will, and not in the absence of anxiety, despite it."

Another thing she loves about Don is that he accepts people for who they are. "You don't want to complain around him, and you don't want to be sad," she said, because ordinary problems seem small compared to what Don faces daily. But Don doesn't see it that way. "He allows people to have their own pain, and he never minimizes it."

Keith Fentress, Don's college roommate and fraternity

brother: Initially after Don's injury, "I felt complete shock at how fragile life is. We started rugby at Virginia Tech. Both of us played on the Virginia Tech team. I have a bad knee. I got hurt playing rugby. That happened before Don got hurt. My rugby experience was already trailing off. That made me start thinking when Don got hit, 'That's it.'"

Fentress assisted Don's family with his care during the first year after his injury. "I felt a gaping hole at having to lose a friend in terms of how we related to each other. Don was a big part of my life in college. A best friend. We spent a lot of time together in and outside of school. His house was on my way home to Chesapeake, and I would always be there on my way to and from breaks."

Don went from being a big brother figure in Fentress' life to someone needing help. "As always Don was inspiring. I know some days he didn't feel like that. But for him to open his eyes every day and see what the day had to offer was an inspiration to everyone."

After his marriage in 1990, Fentress moved to Maryland, became the father of two children, and traveled extensively with his company. He hasn't seen Don in person in years but stays in touch through social media. "We all went through so much together," he says of Don's family. "I think the next time we see each other, we would all smile."

Mike Toney, coach, co-captain of James River Rugby Club at the time Don was injured: Toney was one of the first people to reach Don on the field the day of his injury. "Sometimes I feel guilty that Don's suffering is because of me. That I was the one who put him in that spot," says Toney, who asked Don to play the hooker position.

At the time Toney was 28, a few years older than Don. Toney had been involved with rugby since he was 15. When his older brother was killed in a car wreck at 18, his friends in rugby took Toney under their wing. "The rugby community is very tight knit. It takes care of its own." Rugby contacts helped him get an electrical apprenticeship, which became his career.

Toney played rugby until he was 45. In all that time, Don was one of the few players he knew who ever got hurt in a scrum.

"There are nights that I cry myself to sleep because I semi-blame myself for Don. But then there are times, I am so proud because of his positive outlook on life. That's such a blessing, knowing that Don has taken life and what it has given him. Don is an example of someone who has nothing from the neck down but everything from the neck up."

Today, Toney is a retired electrician who suffers with bad feet. Don's injury "made me appreciate and enjoy life. Right now, I can't feel my feet, but I'd cut them off if I had to. Things can easily be worse. Every day I'm happy to have what I've got."

Toney and Don communicate occasionally by email.

Pat Grover, a rugby teammate, and one of the first people to get to Don after his injury: More than three decades later, the trauma of Don's injury remains fresh in Grover's mind. When asked to return to that day, he begins to cry softly. Grover was playing fullback, a position on the back line, the farthest away from where Don was playing in the scrum. "They called for me," he says of the team. "Everyone knew I was a volunteer paramedic. They knew I had medical training."

When he reached Don's side, "I knew. The fact that he couldn't move, and he couldn't breathe." His girlfriend at the time, who later became his wife, was at the game, standing by with the rescue squad. She was also a paramedic. Along with her was Phillip Green, a member of the rugby team, who didn't play that day because he had squad duty. "At the time it was encouraged, but not required, to have a rescue squad standing by, but you were supposed to have someone with medical training standing by. It turned out to be very fortunate that we had advanced life support there, because he needed to be intubated because he couldn't breathe."

Grover's girlfriend intubated Don, and he was taken to the hospital. In the meantime, Grover finished playing the match. "I cried for the remainder of the game."

Grover continued to play rugby for another 17 years and has traveled the globe attending U.S. rugby events. He occasionally plays in a 55-plus senior tournament and serves as president of the James River Rugby Club. "It's the only catastrophic injury I was ever directly involved with, but there have been others," he said.

Over the years, the sport has implemented rule changes to make the game and the scrum safer. Today, coaches must take training to become certified. Instead of a single referee, matches require a referee and two touch judges. Officials try to ensure that two sides in a scrum come together in a safe and methodical way with a sequence of calls: crouch, bind, set. The changes are designed to reduce the force of impact, making it safer for hookers and other front-row players.

"In the old days, it was just come together and that was the problem," said Grover. "If you weren't ready and your neck or head was in the wrong position, it's not just three people, it's eight people pushing together."

Grover says he attends the annual golf event and any other fundraiser benefiting Don. "I haven't seen him since the last time he came out to the golf tournament, which has been several years ago."

In terms of the impact on his life: "I have a tremendous amount of respect for him and the way he managed himself after the injury. He didn't blame anyone or anything. He continued his educational and career path and basically concluded that this was his destiny and that he was going to make the best of it. I do regret that I don't see him more than I have. I do think about him a lot and communicate with him on Facebook."

Terry Byrd, a rugby teammate on the field the day Don was injured: After Don's paralyzing injury, "Several guys quit after that season. Our team went from being one of the top teams in the state to No. 5 or 6. It took us a while to rebuild."

Byrd, who played 15 years and had already planned to quit due to his impending marriage, also left. "A lot of the guys were married and had wives. Our numbers definitely dropped."

Going to see Don in the hospital was tough. "It made me appreciate life." Byrd married, had children, and worked as a vice president of a bedding company. Because of his love for the game, Byrd later became a rugby referee and remained active with the club, serving as its historian. He also took a course to become a certified coach, so he could help coach the James River Rugby women's team where his daughter plays. Byrd runs the club's annual golf tournament. He and Don email occasionally.

Part Four

New Hope for Paralyzed People

15

Epidural Stimulation: The Next Big Thing?

S ince Don's injury, the field of spinal cord injury research has taken off. Once considered the graveyard
of neuroscience, it's now a speeding train with momentum
fueled by breakthroughs in science and adaptive technologies. One of the most exciting developments is a new focus
on epidural stimulation.

In 2009, Rob Summers became the first quadriplegic
in the world to be implanted with an epidural stimulator
in his lower spine. Paralyzed from the neck down after a
hit-and-run accident, he welcomed the opportunity to serve
as a pioneer for an experimental therapy because anything
was better than the dire prognosis from his doctors. "I was
told I would never walk again."

Summers, a college athlete at the time of his injury, has
no regrets for signing on as the first research subject in a
program at the University of Louisville (UofL) in Kentucky.
Today, Summers can stand, drive a hand-control car, fly

around the country for speaking engagements and live independently in an apartment with his 75-pound golden retriever, Bear. He still gets around primarily in a wheelchair, but the difference in the quality and independence of his life with epidural stimulation has been transformative.

"Being able to stand up at a bar, stand up at the grocery store to get something off the top shelf, just to be able to actively do things out in the general public … It has allowed me to be able to focus and be in the moment with the people around me, instead of worrying about my next medical issue."

In addition, the stimulator has helped him regain other physical capabilities such as temperature regulation, bowel and bladder control and sexual function. "This is definitely the start of the future for the recovery of spinal-cord injured patients," said Summers. "There will be other things brought in," he adds, but Summers predicts that the spinal cord epidural stimulator will become a building block for the paralyzed much like a good pair of running shoes is to a long-distance runner.

Researchers at UofL, and other medical centers hail epidural stimulation as a historic breakthrough, especially for people like Summers whose injuries are considered "motor complete," with total paralysis below the injury level. In clinical studies, research shows that by applying electrical stimulation to the spinal cord, combined with intense physical therapy, these patients can be retrained to move voluntarily, to stand and take steps, while also seeing recovery in autonomic functions such as blood pressure, cardiovascular health and bowel and bladder control. In one study, two patients learned how to walk again with the aid of walkers.

"There are two things that are landmark changes in our knowledge," said Susan Harkema, a professor of neurological surgery at UofL who is leading a federal clinical trial there on epidural stimulation. "One is that the spinal cord is not simply a conduit to control signals from the brain. It has networks of its own, and it can function in all the capacities that we think of as the brain. The circuitry can learn, it can forget, and it can relearn and make decisions."

In other words, the spinal cord has a brain of its own. A second discovery challenges the long-held notion that spinal cord injuries are complete. "What we are finding, so far, is that when we provide epidural stimulation, people can move voluntarily even though they're considered motor complete. We even had someone who is 39 years post injury who could move voluntarily when the stimulator was turned on," said Harkema, who also serves as associate scientific director for the Kentucky Spinal Cord Injury Research Center.

Harkema was referring to Henry G. Stifel III, a well-known name in spinal cord injury research circles. At 17, an auto accident left him paralyzed from the chest down. His injury in 1982 inspired his parents to start a foundation to boost spinal cord injury research, the precursor to what would later become the Christopher & Dana Reeve Foundation. Stifel, a successful New York banker, is a longtime board member of the foundation, so he was familiar with the UofL trial. In 2020, at 55 years old—nearly 39 years after his accident—Stifel enrolled in the university's epidural stimulation trial because he felt his participation could benefit older SCI patients.

After 160 sessions of epidural stimulation, his chronic low blood pressure improved. Stifel's protocol also included 160 two-hour stand training sessions. By the end of the sessions, he could consistently stand for 10 to 16 minutes when the stimulator was on.

The results surprised Harkema. "I admit we had low expectations of Henry being able to move voluntarily after almost four decades of no movement," she said in a story about the program published in the university's newsletter, *UofL News*. "I was stunned when Dr. Angeli [director of the Epidural Stimulation Program] was able to find stimulation configurations for him to sit independently and move his toes, ankles, knees, and hips ... Importantly, this shows that under the right conditions, recovery can happen even decades after injury."

While that sounds miraculous, Harkema points out that following a spinal cord injury the cord isn't totally destroyed. Thousands of neurons die at the point of breakage, but there are millions of neurons and axons below the break that remain intact. Yet the brain can't transmit signals to them because of damage to the cord. "These axons and neurons can learn, function and communicate," said Harkema. They just need a new pathway so they can connect the signals that normally would go to the brain.

That's where epidural stimulation comes in. The electrical current delivered through a spinal implant stimulates intact neural networks in the spinal cord circuitry. The current amplifies signals from the brain and causes muscle contractions, allowing people to consciously move targeted groups of muscles, which also are being retrained through physical therapy.

This therapeutic approach, known as neuromodulation, represents a departure from past thinking where the focus used to be on nerve regeneration through stem cell and other technologies. To date, there is no standard care to regenerate axons in an injured spinal cord.

Summers' journey with epidural stimulation began in 2009, three years after a car veered off the road and struck him, breaking his neck at the C6 vertebra. The accident occurred at night while Summers was retrieving a gym bag from his parked car. The force of the impact knocked him to the ground where he laid undiscovered until the following morning. The 20-year-old, who pitched for the Oregon State University Beavers, dreamed of playing in the major leagues. His paralysis shattered that dream. Yet the role Summers would go on to play as a guinea pig for an experimental treatment giving new hope to millions of paralyzed people is more far reaching than a 90-mile-per hour pitch.

Following rehabilitation and a search of possible therapies at research facilities around the world, Summers signed up for Harkema's UofL program in 2007. At that time, he had regained some use of his upper limbs through intense physical therapy. After two more years of physical rehabilitation at UofL to see if Summers would recover movement in his lower body without electrical stimulation, doctors implanted a 16-electrode array in the epidural space of his back. A wire connects the array to the stimulator, a small rechargeable device similar to a pacemaker that's operated by a remote control. The stimulator is placed under the skin, usually near the buttocks or abdomen.

Following two weeks of rest after his surgery, researchers turned the stimulator on. Summers recalls feeling a tingling sensation. "At first, I was able to move some." A few days later, "I was able to stand up for the first time in years, independently. At that point, we knew we were on to something."

Fast forward to now. Summers is one of 39 people who have been implanted with an epidural stimulator at UofL as part of various clinical trials. Summers is participating in what is known as the "Big Idea" trial funded by the Christopher & Dana Reeve Foundation. Began in 2017, the six-year trial— approved by the U.S. Food and Drug Administration—is designed for a total of 36 participants; so far 25 people have undergone the surgery. The Big Idea seeks to prove that the therapy is viable and can be moved outside the lab.

"The Big Idea is probably the most exciting thing in

the last decade in the field of spinal cord injury research," said Peter Wilderotter, the longtime CEO and president of the Christopher & Dana Reeve Foundation, who stepped down in April of 2021 after 14 years at the helm.

The foundation's reformation in 2000 under the Reeve name ramped up the spotlight on spinal cord injuries, with actor Christopher Reeve using his Hollywood charisma and connections to lobby for more treatments and interventional therapies. Since its inception in 1982 as the Stifel Family Paralysis Research Foundation, which later became the American Paralysis Foundation before joining forces with Reeve, the foundation has raised and invested nearly $140 million in research, said Wilderotter.

Back in 1996, when Reeve traveled the country giving speeches about the dearth of federal funding for spinal cord injury research, the country was spending about $40 million a year. In recent years, the amount has grown from $70 million to nearly $100 million a year, according to Wilderotter. Some of the most innovative work being done is by the U. S. Department of Defense on behalf of America's 40,000 paralyzed veterans. "It's becoming a hot field," said Wilderotter.

He welcomes the momentum but shies away from the word cure. "We have to educate our consumers a lot more and create a roadmap as to what a cure would look like. We're not going to pick up a newspaper and see the headline, 'Spinal cord injury has been cured,'" he said, "because every injury is different. What we will see is incremental differences."

The foundation's first grant for research on epidural stimulation in the 1980s went to Professor Reggie Edgerton at the University of California, Los Angeles (UCLA). Edgerton began by testing the therapy on rats. Turns out there is a striking similarity between the lower lumbar spinal cord of rats and humans. Edgerton, who has been teaching and conducting research at UCLA for more than 40 years, is director of the school's Neuromuscular Research Laboratory. He was one of this country's earliest experimenters with epidural electrical stimulation to treat the spinal cord injured.

Others in the field, including Harkema, cut their teeth while working for Edgerton. Harkema joined his research lab on a fellowship in 1993. "What we saw was that the spinal circuitry in animals, you can reteach them, whereas humans were much more dependent on the brain," she said. Yet, the experiments got the researchers to thinking that maybe they could see the same results in humans.

By 2011, two years after Summers' implant at UofL, Harkema, along with a team of other researchers including Edgerton, published a case study that appeared in scientific journals, including *The Lancet*. It said epidural stimulation enabled Summers to achieve full weight-bearing standing, with assistance provided only for balance, for 4 to 25 minutes. Researchers also noted locomotor-like patterns when stepping during epidural stimulation. Overall, the authors' interpreted the data to mean that "Task-specific training with epidural stimulation might reactivate previously silent spared neural circuits to promote plasticity. These interventions could be a viable clinical approach for functional recovery after severe paralysis."

In 2014, the Christopher & Dana Reeve Foundation reported on the results of a study on epidural stimulation of four young adult males, including Summers. The foundation's research partners at UofL and UCLA said all four men saw improvements in critical autonomic functions such as temperature regulation, and they could move their toes, feet, and legs on command. Upon announcing the results and the Big Idea fund drive on its website, the foundation said, "This recovery challenged the notion that the spinal cord, once damaged, could never be repaired and signaled an unprecedented breakthrough for the field, as well as new hope for the millions living with paralysis."

Studies on epidural stimulation are underway at other facilities as well, including the Mayo Clinic in Minnesota, the Kessler Institute of Rehabilitation in New Jersey, and in Switzerland.

So far, spinal cord injured participants have been outfitted with off-the-shelf spinal stimulators in use primarily for chronic back pain since the 1960s. Edgerton, Harkema, and others assert that results would be more impressive if spinal stimulators could be customized specifically for spinal cord injury. "It's definitely doable," said Harkema, "if we have the appropriate resources and stakeholders. The technology is clearly there."

No surgery is without risk, especially in the spine. According to the FDA, about 50,000 spinal cord stimulators are implanted annually. The agency has received reports of serious side effects in association with the devices when they're used to treat chronic pain. Over a four-year period between July 27, 2016, and July 27, 2020, the FDA received 107,729 reports including 497 associated with patient death, 77,937 with patient injury, and 29,294 with device malfunction. The most frequently cited patient problems were inadequate relief of pain, pain itself, and infection.

Among the deaths associated with the devices, implanted between November 2005 and July 2020, the FDA said that the average age of the patient was 69, and the deaths occurred with the presence of other comorbidities including malignancy and chronic diseases such as diabetes and heart disease. "The submission of an MDR (medical device report) often does not provide enough information to establish a causal relationship between the device and the reported event," the FDA said in a letter to health care providers in September of 2020. The agency sent the letter to remind providers of the importance of conducting a trial stimulation period with patients to confirm satisfactory pain relief before implanting a stimulator.

To make the device as safe as possible, spinal cord injury researchers are pushing for a more targeted device. A new grant is helping UofL move in that direction. In 2021, it received $7.8 million for a five-year project at the school's Kentucky Spinal Cord Injury Research Center in collaboration with medical device manufacturer Medtronic. The goal is to test software applications for Medtronic's commercially available device, Intellius, modifying what is now a spinal cord stimulator for chronic pain into a more programmable device for paralyzed people.

The work, funded through the National Institutes of Health Brain Initiative, "will promote the safe, long-term use of the therapy in the home and community, allowing people with spinal cord injury to benefit from the discoveries we have made over the past two decades," Harkema said in a statement when the grant was announced.

How quickly spinal cord stimulators tailored for paralyzed people move out of the lab and into commercial markets depends largely on a stamp of approval by the FDA. That won't happen without sound research and reliable data to prove the devices work. Also unclear is whether ventilator-dependent quadriplegics like Don could benefit from epidural stimulation. Currently, participants in clinical trials tend to be young and relatively healthy, [with Stifel an outlier] because it is less risky to test a new treatment on them than on older patients or those who are ventilator dependent.

While scientists toil away, Summers continues his journey of healing. He's on his second epidural stimulator, an updated version implanted in 2018. "New things are happening all the time," he observed. "I'm 15 years into this now, and I've seen an exponential growth and change in what's been available over my paralyzed life. There are so many things out there that are evolving and changing. Everything is going to click into place one day, and we'll witness the recovery of spinal cord injury.

"I don't know if cure is the right word," he adds. "What's interesting is that for a lot of people who have lived life in wheelchairs for a long time, it's the secondary functions—the respiratory, blower/bladder, sexual—those are the first things that people in the chairs want. The stepping, the walking, that's what grabs the headlines, but in reality, it's the independence in all these little things that people want to get back first before they start thinking about the movement things."

16

The Role of Uncle Sam

Many people living with spinal cord injury (SCI) in the U.S. are veterans. So, it should come as no surprise that the federal government is a leading funder of research in the field. Many soldiers suffered their injuries while on active duty, particularly during conflicts in Iraq and Afghanistan from 2000 to 2009.

As part of a response to the high rates of SCI injury, Congress established the Spinal Cord Injury Research Program in 2009. Since then, the Department of Defense has invested more than $200 million into research and development efforts to improve the long-term care of injured soldiers.

Injured vets are sent to the country's system of VA hospitals for care and treatment. Ashraf S. Gorgey sees some of these veterans at Central Virginia VA Health Care System in Richmond, one of the largest of the VA's 25 spinal cord injury treatment centers. As the center's director of SCI research, Gorgey heads up several studies that he said hold great promise for the future.

One of them involves combining the use of a robotic exoskeleton, a battery-powered wearable suit, with epidural stimulation. The Department of Defense has awarded the center a $4 million grant to implant 20 patients over the next four years. The grant came after Gorgey's team published a case study in 2019 about the successful results using this approach with one quadriplegic veteran.

After implanting the man with an epidural stimulator, followed by 12 weeks of training on the exoskeleton, he took 575 unassisted steps. The stimulator helped activate his paralyzed muscles while the exoskeleton strapped to his lower limbs helped him take steps. "I never thought in my life that I would see a person up on their feet who hadn't walked in 15 years," said Gorgey.

The center has used exoskeletons alone to help vets take step-like movements since 2014. "It's like braces," Gorgey says of the hard outer suit that supports and protects a person much like an exoskeleton protects the soft tissue of an animal. Giving someone the ability to walk, even haltingly with assistance from the suit and the use of crutches, is huge for people who have been sitting in wheelchairs for years. "It helps a person improve their level of physical activity. When they get up, they can walk from 60 to 75 minutes in one session," said Gorgey.

Just as it isn't healthy for able-bodied people to sit for long periods, so it goes for the spinal cord-injured who frequently gain weight and develop other medical problems because their lives are so sedentary. An exoskeleton provides greater mobility, and the exercise works muscles, improves circulation and cardiovascular health, and promotes other metabolic benefits.

Combining the two experimental therapies, Gorgey said, may be more practical than using epidural stimulation alone. That's because of the intensive rehabilitation now required to improve locomotion prior to implanting an epidural stimulator. The physical training takes time and is staff intensive, he notes. The use of an assistive-walking device reduces training time.

In the past, Gorgey says price has been one of the biggest hurdles for commercial use of exoskeletons, with suits costing $70,000 to $80,000 a piece. As more large manufacturers get in the game, he expects the price to drop to $30,000 to $35,000, still pricey but hopefully within reach if Medicaid and private insurers can be brought on board.

Gorgey, who has published 120 peer-reviewed articles on some of his studies, is also a professor at the Department of Physical Medicine and Rehabilitation at VCU. He began working in the field of spinal cord injury in 2005. "What drives me is that every day we are learning something new...I believe that the field will be skyrocketing with a lot of hope for more interventional clinical trials that will help people with SCI."

Even entrepreneurs like Elon Musk are tinkering with new technologies. Neuralink, a company founded by Musk in 2016, is developing an implantable brain chip that could record and decode electrical signals from the brain. Theoretically the device would serve as a connection between the brain and technology, allowing someone with paralysis to use a computer or phone directly with their brain. The futuristic brain computer interface project has become mired in controversy, however, after a national physicians group sued Neuralink over harm it alleges monkeys suffered during testing of the technology.

The biggest mistake the spinal cord injury field has committed in the past, said Gorgey, is looking for a one-way solution to cure the mystery of the spinal cord. "It won't be one solution. It has to be a multi-interventional way to cure SCI, because you're talking about a system composed of sensory and motor factors and many other things. It's like a puzzle. Each patient is a different puzzle. That's what limits our understanding."

As medicine, neuroscience and engineering converge in this new frontier, Don wonders if the discoveries will help someone like him with an older SCI.

"It will apply to people with complete injury," says Gorgey. Yet, the higher the injury on the spinal cord, like Don's, the more complex the recovery will be.

The Rehab Hospital of Today: Sheltering Arms Institute

Michael Lowery had never heard of a Hocoma Lo-komat until coming to Sheltering Arms Institute. The robotic medical device helped the 39-year-old relearn how to walk. Lowery injured his neck while weightlifting,

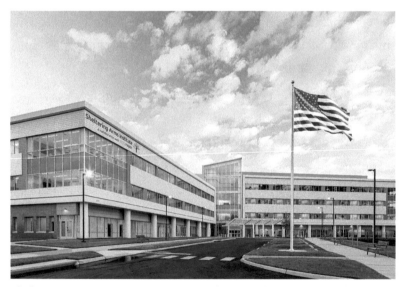

Sheltering Arms Institute in metropolitan Richmond opened in June of 2020 in the middle of the pandemic.

an injury that paralyzed Lowery from the waist down.

The Lokomat made it possible for Lowery to be slipped into a harness, lifted into the air, and lowered onto a treadmill where he could practice walking. The repetitive gait training boosted his confidence and was among several rehabilitative techniques employed in Lowery's recovery.

Upon his arrival, he couldn't move from his wheelchair without assistance. Following several months of physical therapy, Lowery walked out of the hospital with the assistance of a walker.

Welcome to the physical rehabilitation hospital of the 21st century. It's a place, Lowery will tell you, where miracles happen. "At first, when my injury happened, I wanted to kill myself. I didn't want to live anymore because I couldn't move anything." Today, Lowery has returned home to Martinsville, Virginia, where he lives with a high level of independence. "I can get up by myself. Get in the wheelchair by myself. Take a shower. Dress myself."

Getting people back on their feet, literally and figuratively, is one of the hospital's key goals. While all patients can't be restored to pre-injury status, the focus is on maximum recovery so people can live independent and productive lives.

The Lokomat is one of many innovative, state-of-the science technologies at the $95 million, 114-bed, Sheltering Arms Institute that opened in Goochland County, Virginia, in June 2020. It's the first hospital in the U.S. to install the Motek Medical RYSEN, a three-dimensional overground body-weight support system that can be operated from an app. The RYSEN provides therapy for a broad range of locomotive exercises, such as sit-to-stand, walking, turning, and climbing stairs.

The hospital also is seeing success with the EksoNR robotic exoskeleton. The wearable robotic device offers patients upper body support and the chance to practice walking early in the recovery process by retraining the brain and muscles how to walk again. Locomotive specialists can adjust the robot to give more assistance for patients who are weak and less assistance as they become stronger.

Just helping a patient stand upright provides an enormous emotional boost. "For the spinal cord injured, one of the hardest things is to get them up safely," said Joanna Moore, the hospital's spinal cord injury/complex care therapy manager. "We have videos of people hugging their moms and girlfriends while being upright. Some of them haven't been able to stand in months."

In addition to advanced technology, Sheltering Arms Institute offers the latest medical research and clinical care under one roof. The hospital is a collaboration between Virginia Commonwealth University Health System (VCU Health), a teaching hospital that brings the research component, and Sheltering Arms, a nonprofit with a long history of providing clinical care to injured patients throughout Richmond. To create a new hospital focused solely on physical rehabilitation, Sheltering Arms and VCU Health relocated existing beds from three former hospitals, with Sheltering Arms bringing 68 beds and VCU Health, 46.

A recent federal recognition as one of 14 Spinal Cord Injury Model Systems in the country is icing on the cake for the recently opened institute. "There's nothing really like this in the whole mid-Atlantic," said Stephanie Sulmer, the institute's vice president of marketing and business development.

Since opening its doors in June 2021, in the middle of the COVID-19 pandemic, it has become a destination for survivors of strokes, spinal cord injuries, brain injuries, and patients with other neurological disorders such as multiple sclerosis. Patients have come, not only from Virginia, but from nearby states including North Carolina, South Carolina, and Maryland.

Before Sheltering Arms expanded its footprint in Richmond, severely injured patients like Don had to travel out of state to places like the Shepherd Center in Atlanta for physical rehabilitation. While Shepherd is one of the top-ranked, long-term acute care hospitals for rehab in America, "It's tough mentally to be away from family and friends when you're going through rehab," said Don.

Since his injury, physical rehab hospitals have come a long way. Today, there's a big focus on patient-friendly surroundings. Patients have access to private rooms, wide, wheelchair-accessible hallways, automated room shades, and copper-infused sheets that guard against infection.

Aesthetic appeal also is important. Visitors to Sheltering Arms Institute enter through the building's focal point: a four-story glass atrium that floods the lobby with light.

Overhead is a dramatic sculpture recognizing campaign do-nors to the nonprofit, whose foundation raised $50 million to help build the hospital.

The 200,000-square-foot building offers four units: stroke, multi-specialty, traumatic brain injury and spinal cord injury/complex care. Other common diagnoses that send people to Sheltering Arms Institute include multiple joint replacement, amputation, and neuromuscular disor-ders.

Eligible patients must require inpatient hospital treat-ment yet be well enough to participate in three consecutive hours of therapy a day. Besides the main 9,251-square-foot rehabilitation gym on the first floor, there are three satellite gyms on other floors where patients can practice activities of daily living. Each floor is equipped with multiple lounges complete with a kitchen, television, and microwave where families and visitors can spend time with patients. People may also gather in the chapel and dining room.

Patient rooms are spacious and offer flat-screen tele-visions, ensuite bathrooms and overhead lift systems that make it easy for staff to transfer patients from a bed to a wheelchair or the bathroom. Large picture windows overlook a 46-acre, park-like setting. The campus in West Creek Medical Park enjoys a convenient location in metro-politan Richmond, located off Route 288 near Short Pump, a major retail corridor.

The institute employs nearly 400 people, including physical medicine and rehabilitation doctors, nurses; oc-cupational, physical, and respiratory therapists; medical psychologists; care managers; and speech language pathologists. Thanks to the generosity of its foundation, CEO Alan Lombardo says Sheltering Arms Institute provides extra services such as recreational therapy and a chaplain. "We decided to invest in these services to provide a holistic environment," he said.

The hospital takes a three-pronged approach to care: research, technology, and a trans-disciplinary model, with professionals from more than a dozen specialties participating on a patient's care team.

"What is different about this institution is that we have a clinical science team, and they're constantly helping us study the effectiveness of different technologies, connecting us to the latest science," said Dr. Richard Kunz, chief medical officer. This is a significant benefit, he adds, when one considers that typically there's a 17-year gap between the creation of new research and actual implementation of research-based evidence.

In addition to technology, medical science teams in spinal cord research are working on things such as tissue regeneration. "They're trying to reconnect the meaningful connections in an injured spinal cord. That seems to be a little way off," acknowledges Kunz. "But those two things, technology and medical science, are in a race to see what will improve the quality of someone's life the most. Even if you have new connections, there has to be therapeutic shaping in terms of what the spinal cord can do. Technology will probably play a role in that—robotics, virtual reality, basic gaming."

In the meantime, "We do what we can now, and we always move toward the leading edge of science."

Patients work with specialists on how to adapt to their own specific situations. Family members and caregivers may be asked to participate in therapy and training as well, so they can prepare for when their loved one returns home.

An average patient stay is six to nine weeks, said Kemi Fakulujo, the spinal cord injury/complex care nurse manager. Patients on a ventilator may require longer stays.

Also key to the institute's approach is creating a sense of community. During downtime from the physical therapies, social and recreational events give patients a chance to socialize with others. As patients begin to think about reintegrating into the community, they can tap into support groups and peer mentoring. Representatives from 10 organizations, including Sportable, the United Spinal Association, and Brain Injury Association of Virginia, are available to offer direction on everything from how to participate in adaptive sports to finding adaptive housing. Before discharge, care managers craft an after-care plan tailored to each patient that considers caregivers, alterations needed to living environments and training on assistive devices.

Richard Bagby, executive director of the United Spinal Association of Virginia, has mentored many newly injured spinal cord patients. His organization, with more than 400 members in Virginia, also offers individual and family peer mentoring.

Bagby was 24 when a diving accident in 2008 changed

his life. "We were horsing around a swimming pool Labor Day weekend, and we were doing belly flops. The pool wasn't deep enough to jump into." Bagby shot to the bottom and hit his head on concrete, fracturing his C6/C7 vertebrae, which left him paralyzed from the chest down.

A two-sport Division I athlete, Bagby played basketball for Boston University before transferring to the University of Richmond for football. At the time of his accident, he was considering a career in the Marine Corps. Today, he runs the statewide nonprofit, lives independently in a house he built, and drives an adapted car. "Unlike a lot of other injuries, it's very manageable … but you have to do things a little differently to continue doing things," he said.

In the early stages of an injury, people and their families need help in moving past the anxiety. "It is catastrophic. One minute you have your normal as you know it, and the next moment you can't walk, and you can't use the bathroom."

When Bagby counsels with patients at Sheltering Arms Institute, he shares what he has learned and provides an example in the flesh of what's possible. It's easy to feel overwhelmed in the beginning, he says, because so much information is being thrown at people. "It involves learning a new normal. Spinal cord injuries don't change people at their core, who they are as a person. I have found it incredibly rewarding to help folks whether navigating benefit systems or something as mundane as how I close a door after I go through it in a wheelchair."

With places like Sheltering Arms Institute, where medical professionals have put in place the tools and technology to sow recovery, the future looks brighter for the spinal cord injured.

"Those of us in the rehab world shy away from using the word cure, because we always hesitate to provide false hope," said Lombardo. "We think there will be things that are like cures in the future. No one knows when, and no one knows what it will look like. Research is a 10,000-piece puzzle. Maybe we have 2,000 to 3,000 pieces of the puzzle."

One area where advocates are seeing solid success is in the prevention of spinal cord injuries. "Fifty years ago, we were getting more SCIs," said Dr. William McKinley, director of spinal cord injury medicine for VCU Health and a physician on the institute's spinal cord injury unit. "People weren't wearing helmets, seatbelts. Everybody who had a swimming pool had a diving board. You don't see that anymore unless there's a deep end. When you do get an injury, the EMTs [emergency medical technicians] and the hospitals know how to minimize the injury, to keep the back and neck straight, to get you assessed. If you do that, it may keep the injury from being complete."

While it would be gratifying to find a cure, in the meantime, "We have to look for ways we can make improvements for them to function and have quality of life and still maintain good health," said McKinley.

Whether a cure will happen during Don's lifetime is

impossible to predict. If he could move again, the first thing he would do is go fishing. "I always picture myself in a canoe fishing. I think about myself, secluded in a swamp, exploring, and using fishing as an excuse to be exploring."

Hopefully that day will dawn soon.

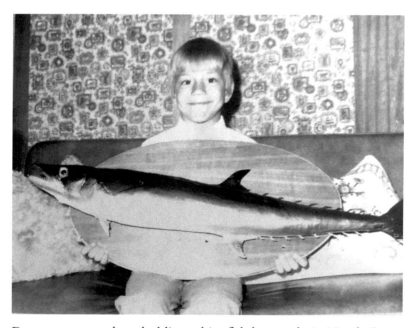

Don, as a young boy, holding a kingfish he caught in North Carolina.

PERSPECTIVE

Science	2
Politics	2
Books	3
Editorials	6

F

Sunday, March 13, 1988

Richmond Times-Dispatch

"I have more good days than bad"

By Paula Crawford Squires
Times-Dispatch staff writer

I gurgles constantly, like the filter on an aquarium. But instead of water, the ventilator pumps air — 10 breaths a minute — into Donald Bridges Jr.'s lungs.

Two units, one on his wheelchair and another beside his bed, keep Bridges alive. He hasn't been able to take a breath since May, when a rugby accident left him paralyzed.

Don, 25, can't feel anything from the neck down. Not the warm sun on his back when he sits outside. Not the soft fur of his stepmother's cat, Blackjack, who frequently naps on Don's feet.

The spinal cord injury that robbed him of movement and sensation didn't impair his mind. Don is still the same bright young man who, before the accident, was a dean's list student in a master's program at the Medical College of Virginia.

He had plans. He and girlfriend Patty Sgueglia had talked of getting married after he received a degree in health administration.

A split-second in a rugby match changed those plans forever. When the ball was put in play, he was in the middle of the surging teams. The impact dislocated his neck and crushed his spinal cord.

Don's reality today and the reality of his family and friends is centered on one thing: keeping him out of a nursing home.

His father, Donald H. Bridges, his stepmother, Ellen, and Ms. Sgueglia have been trained to care for him at home. It's an overwhelming job that has drastically changed the life of this middle-class Chesterfield County family as it tries to cope with Don's catastrophic injury.

[...] disconnection in a telephone line. The spinal cord serves as the body's main [...] carrier, transmitting messages from the brain to the body and back again. After an injury, messages are blocked by damaged nerve fibers. The result: a loss of sensation and movement below the level of the injury.

In Don's case, the damage came at the C3 vertebrae high in his neck. In medical jargon, he is a high-quadriplegic, one of the most severe of spinal cord injuries. "Twenty to 50 percent of the patients with this injury do not survive," said Dr. K. Singh Sahni, a neurosurgeon who treated Don at MCV.

Because the injury severed the nerves to his diaphragm, doctors say there is little chance Don will ever get off the ventilator.

Following his release Jan. 20 from the Shepherd Spinal Center in Atlanta, the Bridgeses had two choices: put Don in a nursing home or care for him themselves. Before the accident, Don lived with his mother, Jutta Bridges, in Colonial Heights. It wasn't feasible for him to return there, Bridges said, since his former wife works and more than one person is needed to care for Don.

Six nursing homes in Virginia accept patients on ventilators. The closest to Richmond is two hours away. Al-

though the state's Medicaid plan would pay for nearly all Don's care, Bridges couldn't bear the thought of putting his only child in a nursing home.

"What I, an individual, his age going to do in a nursing home the rest of his life?We felt a future for him depended on us, what we could do."

Don's injury came at a time when his father, 45, was starting over. This is a second marriage for both Bridges and 36-year-old Ellen. They have been married nearly two years. Mrs. Bridges has no children. That she spends all days now caring for someone, who in many ways is as helpless as an infant, strikes her as ironic.

"Sometimes," she said in a quiet voice, "I wonder if God wasn't saving me for this."

Mrs. Bridges quit a part-time job to help with Don's home care. "To me, this is the only right and natural thing to do. It's not heroic. It's just what needed to be done."

Besides, she adds, "I realized early on that my husband could not live with himself if we didn't make the attempt to keep Don Jr. at home."

She believes home care will speed Don's rehabilitation. "He wants a chance to finish his education and to work. I don't think he would get that in a nursing home."

Don is touched by his family's devotion. "If it wasn't for them, I'd probably just give up."

His immediate goals are to continue graduate studies and to get a job. Mr. and Mrs. Bridges think he has the drive to do it. Their biggest concern now, though, is wondering how they'll pay for a nurse when Don's insurance runs out in May.

Despite the worries, the family hasn't lost its sense of humor. They still find things to laugh about. Don's dry wit

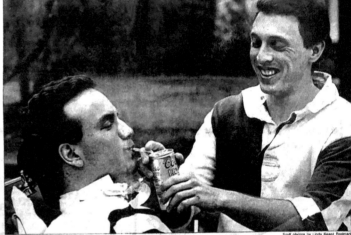

Staff photos by Lindy Keast Rodman

BEST FRIEND — Fraternity brother Keith Fentress of Alexandria, who roomed with Don Bridges at college, visits often. The two friends help each other. Bridges' dry wit keeps Fentress laughing; Fentress helps Bridges with simple tasks like getting a drink.

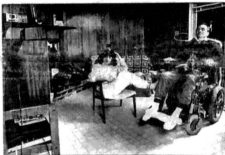

TAKING A BREAK — Patty Sgueglia and Don relax in front of the TV. Ms. Sgueglia took medical training to help care for Don at home. The schedule, on top of her job, proved too taxing

Continued on page 4, col. 1

The *Richmond Times Dispatch* published a story on March 13, 1988, that detailed Don's injury and how family and friends cared for him at home after he became paralyzed. Courtesy *Richmond-Times Dispatch*.

124

"I have more good days than bad"

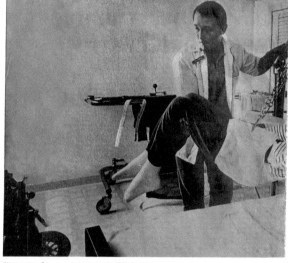

Simply getting Don dressed and moved out of his bed in the morning requires the efforts of stepmother Ellen Br

Continued from first page

is often their inspiration. He recently teased a visitor who mistakenly thought the ventilator supplied him with 10 breaths an hour.

"Ten breaths an hour? I'd be kind of blue, wouldn't I?" he joked.

Laughing in the face of adversity. That is one of the ways Don copes with his injury. That and a refusal to wallow in self-pity.

"I could lay around and feel sorry for myself. That would be the easy thing to do. Many people who have this kind of accident die; I'm still here. There must be a reason. There are still a lot of things I want to do. I'm going to try and do them."

★ ★ ★

7:30 a.m. Don wakes up. Mrs. Bridges and a nurse's aide feed him breakfast while he is still in his hospital bed. Then, Mrs. Bridges cleans the tracheotomy at the base of Don's neck and inserts fresh tubing. She uses sterile gloves to reduce the risk of respiratory infection, one of the greatest concerns of quadriplegics.

8 a.m. The team moves Don from his bed to a shower stretcher. The procedure works like this: The frame of the stretcher is placed on the bed, netting is placed under Don's body and is tied to the frame in eight places. With the help of a lift, the aide raises the frame off the bed a few inches and places it on the stretcher. Don is wheeled into the shower.

Don is wheeled into the shower. Using a spray nozzle, the aide washes his hair and the rest of Don's body. Since he has to be disconnected from the bedside ventilator to be bathed, Ellen manually ventilates Don using a small bag that forces air into his lungs.

8:30 a.m. Don is returned to the bed and reconnected to the ventilator. Ellen shaves him with an electric razor. Next comes one of the day's hardest tasks: dressing. "We have a hard time getting his arms into the shirts," Mrs. Bridges explains. On a good day, the

morning routine takes an hour and a half.

9 a.m. Using a medical lift, the team moves Don from the bed to his wheelchair in much the same way he was moved to the stretcher. What looks like a hammock is placed under Don's 150-pound frame. Chains are hooked to the netting in four places. When the lift is ready, Don is suspended in the air momentarily, before being eased into his chair.

After Don is moved, Mrs. Bridges reconnects him to the ventilator on the base of his wheelchair. When he's in an upright position, she brushes his teeth.

9:15 a.m. At this time, Don has to be suctioned to keep his lungs clear. Quadriplegics can't cough or sneeze, so secretions have a tendency to build up. Mrs. Bridges manually depresses his chest several times to loosen up secretions. Then she inserts a tube into Don's tracheotomy tube and turns on an electric suctioning machine. In the next 24 hours, Don will need to be suctioned four to six times.

9:30 a.m. Don is ready for the day. He spends the rest of the morning watching television and working on his computer. Don operates the computer with a trecnological marvel called a keyboard emulator. This device translates the Morse code and and allows Don to send signals to the computer as if he were at the keyboard. The computer is more than a diversion to Don. It is something over which he has control. He proud shows off a letter he is writing to friend. When he gets the system dow

Don plans to contact some of his professors at MCV to see if he can resume taking courses with the help of the computer.

For Don, running a computer is easier than talking. Since he must wait for the ventilator to give him a breath, his speech is halting. His voice couldn't be heard at all if a cuff wasn't let down on the tracheotomy tube allowing air to pass over his vocal cords. When he is manually ventilated with an bag, as he frequently was during interviews for this story, he speaks normally.

12:00 p.m. Don takes medication to prevent muscle spasms and eats lunch. He is fed by a licensed practical nurse Lois Hogeman. He can eat most anything and has a healthy appetite.

Some days Don has visits from friends. Keith Fentress, who roomed with Don at Virginia Polytechnic Institute and State University and is a fraternity brother, comes often. He also took the medical training and helps the family with Don's care wherever he comes.

Fentress' greatest contribution to his friend's well-being, however, is his ability to make him laugh. He surprises Don with exotic foods like ham and pineapple pizza. And he likes to rehash old times.

The two recently regaled a visitor with tales of practical jokes pulled on unsuspecting fraternity brothers — shaving cream-in-the-face sort of gags. Don shot his friend a warning look. "Don't say too much. There are some things we wouldn't want repeated in the newspaper," he said with a smile.

1 p.m. On Monday, Wednesday, and Friday, physical therapist Lynn Eddy comes to exercise Don's muscles. To prevent stiffness, Ms. Eddy moves each of Don's joints in every direction. They concentrate on exercises to strengthen his neck.

"Push, roll forward. C'mon, c'mon," she encourages as Don moves his neck away from the headrest of the wheelchair. He grimaces as he goes through the counts.

Before the injury, Don was a disciplined athlete. He ran 20 miles a week, lifted weights regularly and was a member of the James River Rugby Football Club.

2 p.m. On nice days, Don goes outside. He drives his wheelchair on the concrete drive beside the family home. By blowing into a mouth straw, he directs air through a tube to the chair's control unit. Using a series of sips and puffs, he can make the chair go, stop, recline.

He spends the rest of the afternoon working on the computer, watching videos or using his new electric sip-and-puff page turner. Don is thrilled to be able to read again. He plans to

ROLL-IN SHOWER — A stretcher, left, allows Don to be wheeled into a 6- by 8-foot shower that was added to Brighton Green home.

reread his favorite book, Joseph Conrad's "The Heart of Darkness."

6 p.m. By this time, Bridges, a supervisor in the purchasing department at Virginia Power, returns home. Ellen cooks dinner upstairs and brings it downstairs so the family can eat together.

Don has never seen the upstairs of his parents' home. The family looked into the cost of an outside elevator lift. The price tag of $4,800 was prohibitive. After dinner, Ellen cleans up and Bridges visits with his son.

9:30 p.m. The couple get Don ready for bed. They suction him and catheterize his bladder. He is moved from the wheelchair to the bed.

The Bridgeses sleep upstairs. If Don needs help during the night, he calls for them over an intercom. If the ventilator malfunctions, an alarm system will sound downstairs and in the upstairs bedroom. On many nights, Bridges or his wife gets up at least once to suction Don's lungs and to turn him to prevent bedsores.

★ ★ ★

The first six weeks Don was home, Ms. Sgueglia, 23, served as his nightcare person. She cooked for him, kept him company and got up with him during the night.

After putting in a full day's work in the marketing department of the American Historical Foundation, Ms. Sgueglia said the night schedule proved too exhausting. She moved out of the house. But she hasn't forgotten about Don. "I plan to stay in touch," she said.

The couple first met on a blind date on Feb. 15, 1986. Ms. Sgueglia feels more sad than bitter about Don's accident. "It's a lot to accept. It's hard to see someone you love like this."

In addition to scrapping the couple's marriage plans, the accident has had another, perhaps even more profound, effect on Ms. Sgueglia. "My sense of priorities has changed."

"I get pretty impatient with what people think is so important," she explained, "like having to run off and plan their wedding for six months. It makes me laugh. But then again, that's important to them. If I was never in this situation, I would still think that, you know. . . ." Her voice trailed off.

Don still keeps her picture on the table by his bed.

Immediately after the accident, there were times when he thought he would be better off dead. "I had visions of myself lying in a bed the rest of my life on a respirator not being able to do anything," he said. "Now, there are a lot of things I can do. . . . I have more good days than bad."

Although he tries to dwell on the positive, he misses things other people take for granted. Like privacy. "I used to love nothing more than to slip off to the library at school for five to six hours to do schoolwork and have some time to myself."

What does he miss the most? The simplest of human motions.

"It would be nice to wake up in the morning, throw the covers off and get up out of bed."

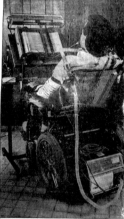

Staff photo by Lindy Keast F

MODERN TECHNOLOGY — Don reads with the h an electric page turner activated by a mouth straw.

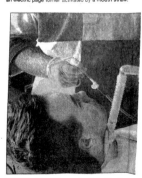

CLEARING HIS LUNGS — Quadriplegics pirato can't cough or sneeze and are prone to res- Don is

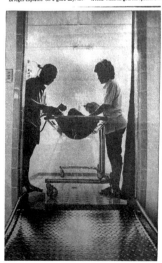

Staff photo by Lindy Keast Rodman

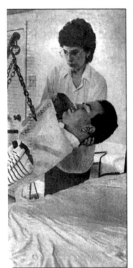
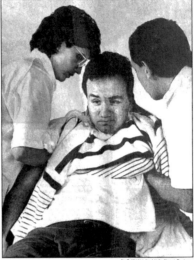

An expensive alternative

By Paula Crawford Squires
Times-Dispatch staff writer

When Donald and Ellen Bridges decided to care for his paralyzed son in their own home, they learned how expensive a catastrophic injury can be.

Mrs. Bridges estimates the couple spent or borrowed $35,000 preparing for the homecoming of Donald Bridges Jr., a quadriplegic who breathes with the assistance of a ventilator.

They sold their three-story town house, bought a home in the Brighton Green subdivision of Chesterfield County, modified its lower level to make it wheelchair accessible and purchased a $19,000 van with a wheelchair lift. Home modifications, which included the widening of doorways and construction of a 6-by-8 foot shower, cost about $11,500.

One of the biggest expenses the Bridgeses will face soon is private nursing care. Because Don is disabled, Medicaid provides a nurse's aide six hours a day, five days a week. The aide helps Don with basic activities such as bathing and dressing, but is not trained to perform medical tasks he needs. Mrs. Bridges is frequently the one who suctions his lungs and monitors the ventilator that keeps Don alive.

Funds from a small student insurance policy Don had at the time of his accident have paid for a nurse, eight hours a day, during the week. The nurse enables Mrs. Bridges to leave the house long enough to run errands.

In May, the insurance money runs out. If additional funds can't be found, Bridges said, "Ellen will become virtually housebound."

The annual cost of providing a daytime nurse during the week, not counting weekends or holidays, would be about $28,000. This figure is based on the $13.75-per-hour private nursing rate charged to the insurance policy now.

Bridges earns about $60,000 a year, including his salary from a job at Virginia Power and an Army pension. Don receives a monthly $340 supplemental security check.

After he pays the family's bills and tries to get some of the equipment he feels will make Don's life easier, Bridges said, "We don't have anything left."

What galls Mrs. Bridges is that Medicaid laws will not allow the family to apply the $7-an-hour allotment for the aide to a nurse.

In a letter to Sen. John W. Warner, R-Va., she spilled out her frustrations: "Prior to Don's injury, it would have been hard for me to believe that an average upper-middle-class family could find itself in a predicament such as ours," she wrote. "All we want is to keep Don out of a nursing home and give him the best possible quality of life. . . . Will we have to bankrupt ourselves to do it?"

A bill pending in the House could help families like Don's. Proposed by Rep. Claude Pepper, D-Fla., it calls for increased Medicare funds to cover long-term home health care for the elderly and working-age people disabled by illness or accidents.

Efforts are also under way in Virginia to set aside more state money for residential care of people who otherwise would be in more-expensive nursing homes.

Ray T. Sorrell, director of the state Department of Medical Assistance Services, sympathizes with the Bridgeses' plight, but says nothing can be done, since the state's Medicaid plan does not cover private nursing care in the home.

He points out that the plan has spent about $151,000 so far on Don, picking up the tab for his four-month stay at a rehabilitation center and for a portion of his wheelchair and other medical equipment.

He concedes, however, that the couple is saving the state money by caring for Don at home. Charlotte C. Carnes, manager of community-based care for the state Medicaid plan, said if the Bridgeses put Don in a nursing home, the cost of his care would run $42,500 a year.

The state and federal Medicaid programs would split that amount about 50-50; Don would pay a small fee.

Mr. the Mrs. Bridges don't think Don, 25, would be happy in a nursing home. They're trying to raise funds for nursing care. Mrs. Bridges has sent letters to area businesses and addressed civic clubs. Don's former schoolmates at the Medical College of Virginia have set up a trust fund at Signet Bank called "Help Don Succeed."

So far, the efforts have resulted in about $25,000 worth of contributions. Much of that money has been spent, however, on equipment that Medicaid wouldn't cover.

At this point, the family doesn't know what else it can do. In its struggle to keep a loved one at home. "There are a lot of uncertainties. . . . It gets scary sometimes," Bridges says.

His wife agrees. "I still wonder sometimes if I'm equal to this on a long-term basis. I hope to God I am."

Staff photos by Lindy Keast Rodman

Injury focuses attention on rules

On the average, it happens once a year during rugby matches played in this country: An accident leaves someone paralyzed. That's the figure given by Dr. John C. Gordon, medical director of the Eastern Rugby Union in Baltimore.

While rugby as a sport doesn't result in the highest number of spinal cord injuries, rugby officials are considering rule changes to make the game safer.

Dr. John Nixon, honorary secretary of the U.S. Rugby Football Union, said an injury suffered by a Richmond area resident last year helped focus attention on the need for one change that has already been made.

Donald Bridges Jr. of Colonial Heights, while playing the hooker position, dislocated his neck during a scrum at a rugby match May 2. The spinal cord injury left him paralyzed from the neck down.

This injury and others like it in recent years made rugby officials take a hard look at the scrum, a formation used to put dead balls back into play. It entails throwing the ball in between two walls of opposing players, eight men to a side.

In the past, Dr. Nixon noted, some scrums "would charge into each other like two stags." Since rugby players lock their arms around one another's shoulders during this formation, people are pressed together, with hundreds of pounds of weight bearing down on them.

This is particularly true for hook-

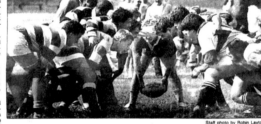

U.S. rugby union officials are considering rule changes to make the scrum formation safer.

Staff photo by Robin Layton

ers, who are trying to kick the ball out, and the two players next to them. They are in the front row and have people pushing in on them from all sides. If they lose their balance, their arms aren't free to break a fall.

In October, the football union approved a rule change that Dr. Nixon believes "takes the aggression out of the initial impact when that scrimmage goes down." Now teams must crouch, then touch, then engage.

Dr. Nixon, a cardiologist at the Medical College of Virginia and a former rugby referee, says more

changes affecting the scrum are in the works.

Among the 8,000 to 10,000 new spinal cord injuries reported a year, 47.7 percent are caused by car accidents, 20.8 percent by falls, 14.6 percent by acts of violence such as gunshot wounds and 14.2 percent by sports accidents.

The rest can't be put into a specific category, according to figures provided by the National Institute on Disability and Rehabilitation Research in Washington.

Dr. Lyle J. Micheli, director of

sports medicine at Harvard Children's Hospital in Boston, says studies have shown that football, which in this country is played by thousands more people than rugby, is the riskiest organized sport in terms of catastrophic head and neck injuries.

Last year, the National Head and Neck Injury Registry at the University of Pennsylvania, which tracks football injuries, reported six accidents that caused players to become quadriplegics. In earlier years, before rules were changed about tackling with the top of the helmet, the number was higher. — SQUIRES

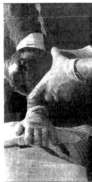

infections. To keep his lungs clear, suctioned several times a day.

Staff photo by Lindy Keast Rodman

Medical advances offer new hope

Years ago, doctors wouldn't even talk about a cure for paralysis. Victims of spinal cord injuries were told nothing could be done. They would spend the rest of their lives in a wheelchair.

Today, there is still no cure, but encouraging advances have been made. Experiments in rats and monkeys are offering new hope that people with spinal injuries may one day regain some use of their paralyzed limbs.

The main obstacle to finding a cure — damaged spinal nerves in the central nervous system don't grow back — hasn't changed, but the approach has.

At Case Western University in Cleveland, Jerry Silver, associate professor of developmental genetics, has been able to regenerate crushed nerves and to restore reflexes in adult rats.

At the University of Florida, surgeons are transplanting spinal cells in monkeys. The experiments involve filling lesions in the monkey's injured spinal cord with transplanted embryonic spinal cord cells.

University spokesman Larry Lansford said it remains to be seen whether the monkey's brain will be able to send impulses to nerve cells over the grafted connections. Testing on humans is still a long way off.

The Medical College of Virginia, in conjunction with McGuire Veterans Administration Medical Center here, is using electrical stimulation to relieve muscle spasticity, a common problem for paralyzed people. So far, electrodes have been implanted in 25 patients. — SQUIRES

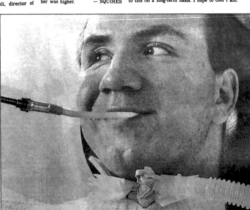

Staff photo by Lindy Keast Rodman

Quadriplegic conquers with computer

By Paula Crawford Squires
Times-Dispatch staff writer

Two weeks ago, Donald Bridges Jr. didn't think he was going to graduate with his class. Papers had piled up and he was running out of time.

But, as is usually the case with Bridges, who is paralyzed from the neck down, perseverance triumphed over self-doubt.

So, there he was yesterday, joking with classmates during a reception for master's degree recipients in the garden of the Valentine Museum.

When the class gathered for a picture, Bridges waited while everyone lined up on the garden steps. Then, he carefully moved his breath-con-trolled wheelchair into place.

"I just feel so proud," said his father, Donald Bridges Sr.

"We made it, the first part of the journey," said the elder Bridges' wife, Ellen.

"For him to have achieved what he has achieved, I think it's an inspiration to other people," added Bridges' mother, Jutta Jordan-Shahin.

Bridges himself was more low key. "I'm relieved," he said.

He also expressed thanks to his family, friends and the faculty and staff at MCV. "A lot of people have shown support and had a hand in this along the way."

Yesterday was a history-making day at the Medical College of Virginia. Not just because a 27-year-old quadriplegic, who breathes with the assistance of a ventilator, completed his education against great odds.

But because he did it with a class of new-age learners.

Bridges and 20 other students were recognized for being the first class to complete an innovative program of computerized instruction that educators say is a prototype for the future.

Designed for mature, working professionals, the two-year Executive Program in health administration allows people in health care professions to

Continued on page 2, col. 3

Quadriplegic, 27, uses computer to conquer odds

Continued from first page

return to graduate school via the computer. An advantage, noted program coordinator Dennis D. Pointer, is that students don't have to live within driving distance of MCV.

A personal computer and modem gain them access to MCV's computer, where assignments are given and reviewed. "There's really nothing like this anywhere in the commonwealth," noted Pointer.

MCV's program is the second in the country. Dr. Gary L. Filerman, president of University Programs in Health Administration and the keynote speaker during yesterday's ceremony, said, "The world is moving toward this form of delivery in higher education."

Many of the students in the program were from out-of-state, but were in Richmond last week finishing up course work. That's why MCV decided to hold the reception and a ceremony at the Lyons Building in lieu of a formal graduation.

At Virginia Commonwealth University, of which MCV is a division, graduations are held only in May, August and December. The mock degrees given out yesterday will be followed up with official degrees that will be mailed in August.

Besides the computer work, students were required to attend intensive on-campus seminars six times during the two years. The seminars were videotaped for Bridges, although he did participate last week in final on-campus seminars. Instead of written exams, faculty assistants traveled to Bridges' home in Chesterfield County and allowed him to orally respond to test questions. These were the main adjustments made for Bridges, who had the same requirements and deadlines for papers and projects as everyone else.

Bridges began work on his graduate degree in 1987 to further a career in health management. He'd previously worked at a local hospital. In May of that year, an injury during a rugby match left him paralyzed and unable to breathe on his own.

After undergoing rehabilitation at the Shepherd Spinal Center in Atlanta, Bridges returned to Chesterfield to live with his father and stepmother.

They bought a home and remodeled it extensively so he wouldn't have to live in a nursing home. Bridges returned to graduate school in January 1988 when MCV began the program that happened to be in his field.

The technological marvel that enables Bridges to run a computer is called a magic wand keyboard. The size of a postcard, it's mounted on a flexible arm attached to Bridges' wheelchair and is electronically connected to his PC computer.

The keyboard has all the

tronically registered as key strokes on the computer.

The process is slow, but enables Bridges to do his own typing. "If I'm on a roll, I can type 20 to 25 words a minute," he says.

The keyboard and a modem were purchased for Bridges by the State Department of Rehabilitation Services. Teresa Wingold, who has served as Bridges rehabilitative counselor since 1988, expressed pride in Bridges' achievement.

"A number of quadriplegics finish college, but in his case with the ventilator and 24-hour attendant care, that makes it a little more complicated," she said.

Pointer, too, who had Bridges as a student both before and after his accident, praised Bridges' drive. "He brought a unique contribution to the program. First, as a person, and second, because of his interest in the disabled and handicapped."

Now that he's finished, Bridges is anxious to find a job. "I'd like to get into health policy analysis and research," he said.

Eventually, his goal is to start a home for ventilator-dependent quadriplegics, so they would have options other than living with families or going into nursing homes.

Unlike other graduates, Bridges has another unique concern: He can't make too much money. If he does, he

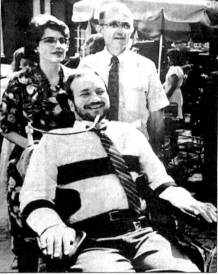
Staff photo by Don Long

ACHIEVEMENT — Donald Bridges Jr. is joined by his father and stepmother at a reception at the Valentine Museum.

won't be eligible for Medicaid, which helps pay for medical supplies and some of his at-home nursing care.

Although programs are in place that allow severely disabled people

like Bridges to earn more than what is generally permitted, his income will always have to be curtailed if he wants to remain eligible for the benefits.

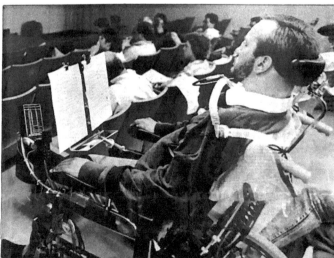

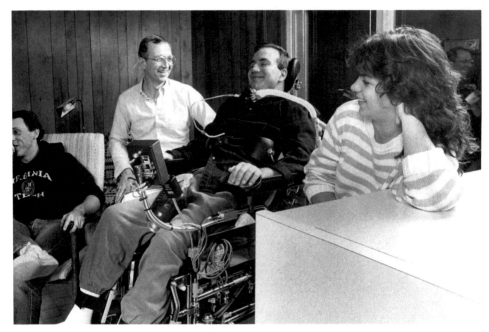

Don relaxing at home in 1988 with (from left) friend, Keith Fentress; dad, Donald Bridges Sr.; and girlfriend, Patty Sgueglia.

Page 127: A front-page story in the June 10, 1990, edition of the *Richmond Times-Dispatch* covered Don's graduation from a master's degree program in health administration at what was then the Medical College of Virginia. Courtesy *Richmond Times-Dispatch*.

ACKNOWLEDGMENTS

The idea for this book came after reading the novel, *Me Before You*, by Jojo Moyes. The fictional tale, set in England, tells the story of a wealthy young businessman who is paralyzed from the neck down after being hit by a motorcycle. It's a painful transition for Will Traynor, a financial wheeler dealer and extreme sports enthusiast. He falls in love with his caregiver, but even that relationship is not enough to dissuade him from choosing euthanasia over life in a wheelchair.

The book intrigued me because I knew someone in real life who had a dramatically different outlook. Donald Bridges Jr. dislocated his neck playing rugby in 1987. He decided early on to do the best he could in life, despite being paralyzed from the neck down and dependent upon a ventilator to breathe. Don has lived with his paralysis for 35 years.

After leaving magazine journalism in 2018, I suggested doing a book on Don's life and how he has persevered. I want to express my deepest thanks to Don for trusting me to tell his story.

Don made himself available for interviews over a period of several years and allowed me to share in his life. I am indebted to his family members, friends, and former rugby teammates who spoke with me about Don's injury and how it affected their lives.

My gratitude also goes to his long-time friends, Chet and Tammy Willis. They have been part of Don's journey from the beginning, and they gladly shared their memories and observations over the years.

Another person who was hugely helpful was Angela Scharmer, Don's now retired head nurse. She explained the nuances of caring for a quadriplegic and the health dangers faced by paralyzed people.

The book was deeply enriched by interviews with staff at Sheltering Arms Institute in Goochland County. Stephanie Sulmer, vice president for marketing and business development, set up not one, but two tours—one for me, and another for Don—so we could visit this modern and innovative hospital where the latest in therapeutic care and technologies are available to the spinal cord injured. Executives, therapists, and nursing staff gladly shared their time to help me understand the workings of a modern rehabilitation hospital.

The Richmond region of Virginia is fortunate to be home to Sheltering Arms Institute and the Central Virginia VA Health Care System, one of the largest of the Veteran Affairs' 25 spinal cord injury treatment centers. Thanks to Ashraf Gorgey, the center's director of spinal cord injury research, for giving me a tour, showing me an exoskeleton, and sharing his team's exciting research on some of the new approaches to assist people with spinal cord injuries.

I am also deeply indebted to the visionary researchers who acquainted me with the new frontier that is spinal cord injury research today. Susan Harkema, a professor of neurological surgery at the University of Louisville, walked me through federal trials she is leading for epidural stimulation, one of the most promising new treatments. Putting a human face on this therapy was Rob Summers, who gave an interview on the challenges of being the first quadriplegic in the world to be implanted with an epidural stimulator.

My unending gratitude goes to my husband, the late Dean Squires. He was my first reader, offering sound counsel. And he was always a champion of my dreams. Thank you, Dean, for your encouragement during the writing of this project. I could not have done it without you.

The unconditional love and support from our daughters, Jessie Colwell and Katie Shortlidge, also inspired this book. Thank you for being the muses who always encourage Mom.

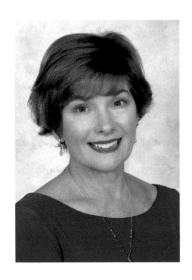

ABOUT THE AUTHOR

Paula C. Squires is an award-winning journalist. Based in Virginia, she has reported for the *Virginian-Pilot* and the *Richmond Times-Dispatch*, where she also served as the consumer affairs columnist. As former managing editor of *Virginia Business* magazine, Squires traveled the state interviewing top business leaders and covering major events. Her stories have won state and national awards, and her work has appeared in regional magazines and the *Associated Press*. Squires is the author of a history of the Virginia Realtors Association, the state's largest professional trade association. A graduate of Radford University, she lives in Midlothian, Va.

website: www.paulasquires.com

Notes on Sources

Introduction

1. Headline and quotation referenced in newspaper story: Paula Crawford Squires, "I have more good days than bad," *Richmond Times-Dispatch*, March 13, 1988.

Prologue

2. Tour of Sheltering Arms Institute, Goochland County, Virginia, with Donald Bridges Jr. on May 24, 2021.

Chapter One: 'Organized Mayhem'

3. Don Bridges Jr., interviews with author, from October 2018 to April 2022, Chesterfield County, Virginia.

4. Mike Toney, interview with author, August 24, 2019, Chesterfield County, Virginia.

5. Reference to sport being described as "organized mayhem": Phillip Brents, "Brave New World: Rugby Starting to Attract Attention," *The Star News*, April 26, 2018. Thia Markson, Lorraine LoBiano, Organized Mayhem: The Story of the B.A.T.S Rugby Club. A 2019 documentary about one of the country's most successful amateur rugby clubs, the Bay Area Touring Side, based in San Francisco.

6. Patty Sgueglia, telephone interview with author, January 27, 2022.

Chapter Two: The Scrum

7. Terry Byrd, interview with author, August 27, 2019, Chesterfield County, Virginia.

8. Pat Grover, interview with author, August 26, 2019, Chesterfield County, Virginia.

9. Patty Sgueglia, author interview.

10. Reference to physical force exerted by players in a rugby scrum: Tod Leonard, "The Art of the Scrum: Legion players explain rugby's mysterious melee," *Baltimore Sun*, June 7, 2019.

Chapter Three: Calm Before the Storm

11. Ellen Eggerding, (formerly Ellen Bridges) telephone interview with author, June 3, 2019.

12. Donald Bridges Sr., interviews with author, December 8, 2019; November 4, 2021, Chesterfield County, Virginia.

13. Patty Sgueglia, author interview.

14. Dr. Kevin Keller, telephone interview with author, October 10, 2019.

15. Don Bridges Jr., author interview.

16. Christopher Reeve's cause of death: "Even Superman Couldn't Win Battle With Pressure Ulcers," *Science Daily*, August 23, 2006.

Chapter Four: Miracle Man?

17. Ashraf Gorgey, interview with author, October 30, 2019, Central Virginia VA Health Care System, Richmond, Virginia.

18. Susan Harkema, telephone interview with author, January 21, 2021.

19. Kemi Fakulujo, author interview, May 24, 2021, Shelter-

9

ing Arms Institute, Goochland County, Virginia.

20. Dr. William McKinley, telephone interview with author, September 23, 2020.

21. Christopher Reeve's quote comes from the book jacket, *Still Me*, by Christopher Reeve, Random House, New York, 1998.

22. Don Bridges Jr., author interview.

23. Chet Willis, interviews with author, August 25, 2019; Feb. 15, 2022, Chesterfield County, Virginia.

24. Steve Smith, interview with author, July 28, 2019, Chesterfield County, Virginia.

25. Patty Sgueglia, author interview.

26. Angela Scharmer, telephone interview with author, January 24, 2022.

Chapter Five: Rehabilitation

27. Ellen Eggerding author interview.

28. Don Bridges Jr., author interview.

29. National Spinal Cord Injury Statistical Center website, Facts and Figures 2021, www.nscisc.uab.edu.

30. Statistics on number of people in America living with paralysis come from Policy Data Brief, Christopher & Dana Reeve Foundation.

31. Figure on number of people in Virginia receiving spinal cord injury care in Virginia, Ashraf Gorgey, author interview.

32. Don Bridges Sr., author interview.

Chapter Six: Homecoming

33. Ellen Eggerding, author interview.

34. Don Bridges Sr., author interview.

35. Tammy Willis, interview with author, August 25, 2019, Chesterfield County, Virginia.

Chapter Seven: Starting Over

36. Ellen Eggerding, author interview.

37. Don Bridges Jr., author interview.

38. Information on Don's daily care and routine shortly after injury, Paula Crawford Squires, *Richmond Times-Dispatch*, "I have more good days than bad," March 13, 1988, Perspective Section, 1.

39. Don Bridges Sr., author interview.

40. Don Bridges Jr., author interview.

41. Patty Sgueglia, author interview.

Chapter Eight: Back to School

42. Don Bridges Jr., author interview.

43. Description of electronic graduate program in health administration at the Medical College of Virginia in 1988, Paula Crawford Squires, "Linkup Is Paralysis Victim's Ticket Back," *Richmond Times-Dispatch*, September 4, 1988.

44. Description of Don's graduate day and quotations from people who attended the ceremony, Paula Crawford Squires, "Quadriplegic Conquers With Computer," *Richmond Times-Dispatch*, June 10, 1990.

Chapter Nine: Work

45. Keith Fentress, telephone interview with author, February 11, 2022.

46. Figures on earnings allowed for people on social security disability insurance come from Social Security website, www.ssa.gov.

47. Don Bridges Jr., author interview.

Chapter Ten: Spiritual Hunger

48. Don Bridges Jr., author interview.

49. Steve Smith, author interview.

50. Observations of church service come from a visit to the Brandermill Ward, The Church of Jesus Christ of Latter-day Saints, July 20, 2019, Chesterfield County, Virginia.

51. Aaron Gregory, telephone interview with author, October 15, 2020.

Chapter Eleven: Marriage, On His Own

52. Newspaper account of Don's romance, marriage, and fatherhood: Bill Lohman, "A Dad at Last: Instant Family Fulfills a Dream," *Richmond Times-Dispatch*, June 18, 2000.

53. Don Sr., author interview.

54. Chet Willis, cost of home renovation, author interview.

Chapter Twelve: The Help

55. Information about pay for private duty nurses for Medicaid patients comes from telephone interview with

Rebecca Stricklin, care management specialist, Department of Medical Assistance Services, August 24, 2020.

56. Don Bridges, Jr., author interview.

57. Figure on number of people in Virginia receiving Medicaid waiver benefits comes from Stricklin interview.

58. Angela Scharmer, interview with author, November 11, 2021, Chesterfield County, Virginia.

59. Neana Hines, interview with author, December 16, 2021, Chesterfield County, Virginia.

Chapter Thirteen: The Power of Community

60. Terry Byrd, author interview.

61. Chet Willis, memo to author, February 15, 2022.

62. Chet and Tammy Willis, author interview.

63. Don Bridges Jr., author interview.

64. Dr. Kevin Keller, interview with author, November 7, 2019, Chesterfield County, Virginia.

65. Steve Smith, author interview.

66. The quote from Brooke Ellison's commencement speech comes from her book: *Miracles Happen, One Mother, One Daughter, One Journey*, 2001, Hyperion, New York.

Chapter Fourteen: Ripple Effect: How an SCI Affects Family and Friends

67. Don Bridges, Sr., author interview.

68. Ellen Eggerding, author interview.

69. Patty Sgueglia, author interview.

70. Keith Fentress, author interview.

71. Mike Toney, author interview.

72. Pat Grover, author interview.

73. Terry Byrd, author interview.

Chapter Fifteen: Epidural Stimulation: The Next Big Thing?

74. Rob Summers, telephone interview with author, September 1, 2020.

75. Susan Harkema, telephone interview with author, January 12, 2021.

76. Betty Coffman, "New York man with paralysis stands 39 years after injury thanks to UofL's spinal cord research," *UofL News*, Feb. 1, 2022.

77. Peter Wilderotter, telephone interview with author, July 30, 2020.

78. Christopher Reeve cited the $40 million federal funding figure in a speech to the Democratic National Convention, August 26, 1996.

79. Explanation of results of epidural stimulator implant, *The Lancet*, Volume 377, Issue 9781, P1938-1947, June 4, 2011.

80. Brief summary on results of study on epidural stimulation involving four young adult men comes from Christopher & Dana Reeve Foundation website at www.christopherreeve.org.

81. Reports on side effects in patients when spinal cord stimulators were used to treat chronic pain, Federal Drug Administration website at www.fda.gov.

82. Information on grant for University of Louisville, UofL newsletter, Betty Coffman, "UofL receives $ 7.8 million grant to enhance epidural stimulation technology for individuals with spinal cord injury." March 16, 2021.

Chapter Sixteen: The Role of Uncle Sam

83. Website, Spinal Cord Injury Research Program, Department of Defense, https://cdmrp.army.mil.

84. Ashraf Gorgey, telephone interview, August 24, 2020.

85. *Annals of Clinical and Translational Neurology*, 2020, P259-265. "The feasibility of using exoskeletal-assisted walking with epidural stimulation: a case report study."

Chapter Seventeen: The Rehab Hospital of Today

86. Michael Lowery, author interview, September 10, 2020, Sheltering Arms Institute, Goochland County, Virginia; telephone interview, December 30, 2020.

87. Descriptions of rehabilitation equipment and interviews with Sheltering Arms' executives and nursing personnel come from tours of the facility taken on September 10, 2020, and May 24, 2021.

88. Don Bridges Jr., author interview.

89. Ranking of Shepherd Center as one of 10 best hospitals in U.S. for rehabilitation, *U.S. News & World Report*, Best Hospitals issue, July 27, 2021.

90. Richard Bagby, telephone interview with author, September 28, 2020.

91. Dr. William McKinley, author interview.

92. Don Bridges Jr., author interview.

93. Stories about Don that appeared in the *Richmond Times-Dispatch* were reproduced with permission of the newspaper.

Bibliography

Published Works

Cerda, Ray Jr., *The Life I Didn't Expect, Facing Adversity and Winning*, 2019.

Ellison, Brooke, and Jean, *Miracles Happen, One Mother, One Daughter, One Journey*, Hyperion, 2001.

Ellison, Brooke, *Look Both Ways*, Small Batch Books, 2021.

Moyes, JoJo, *Me Before You*, Penguin Books, 2012.

Reeve, Christopher, *Still Me*, Random House, New York, 1998.

Christopher & Dana Reeve Foundation, *Paralysis Resource Guide*, Fourth Edition, 2017.

LeGrand, Eric, with Mike Yorkey, *Believe, My Faith and The Tackle That Changed My Life*, William Morrow, an imprint of HarperCollins Publishers, 2012.

Documentary Films

Hunt, Ian A., Reeve, Matthew; Watts, Stuart; directors, Christopher Reeve: *Hope in Motion*. Produced by Alastair Waddington, 2002.

Markson, Thia Markson; LoBianco, Lorraine, directors, *Organized Mayhem: The Story of the B.A.T.S Rugby Club*. 2019.

INDEX

COURAGE

COURAGE